The Path to Stress-Free Nursing Professional Development

50 No-Nonsense Solutions to Everyday Challenges

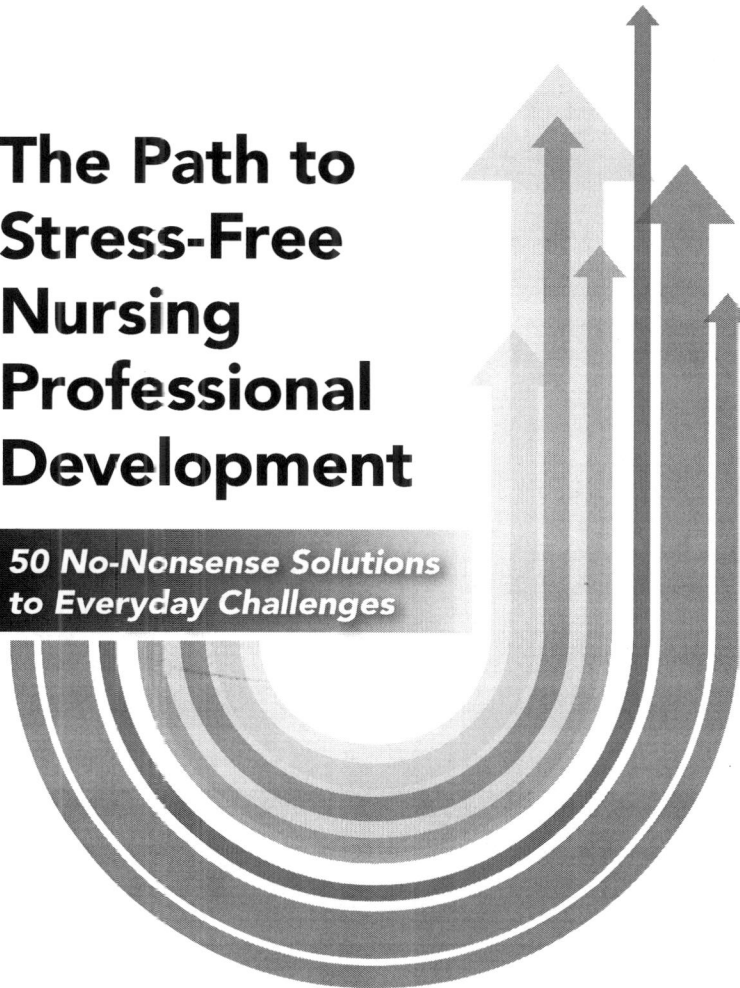

Adrianne E. Avillion, DEd, RN

with contributing author

Barbara A. Brunt, MA, MN, RN-BC, NE-BC

⊢CPro

The Path to Stress-Free Nursing Professional Development: 50 No-Nonsense Solutions to Everyday Challenges is published by HCPro, Inc.

Copyright © 2012 HCPro, Inc

Cover Image © vector-RGB, Shutterstock.

All rights reserved. Printed in the United States of America.   5   4   3   2   1

Download the additional materials of this book at *www.hcpro.com/downloads/10170*.

ISBN: 978-1-60146-930-4

HCPro, Inc., provides information resources for the healthcare industry.

HCPro, Inc., is not affiliated in any way with The Joint Commission, which owns the JCAHO and Joint Commission trademarks.

"MAGNET™, MAGNET RECOGNITION PROGRAM®, and ANCC MAGNET RECOGNITION® are trademarks of the American Nurses Credentialing Center (ANCC). The products and services of HCPro, Inc., and The Greeley Company are neither sponsored nor endorsed by the ANCC. The acronym MRP is not a trademark of HCPro or its parent corporation."

Adrianne E. Avillion, DEd, RN, Author	Mike Mirabello, Graphic Artist
Barbara A. Brunt, MA, MN, RN-BC, NE-BC, Contributing Author	Matt Sharpe, Production Manager
Tami Swartz, Editor	Shane Katz, Art Director
Rebecca Hendren, Associate Editorial Director	Jean St. Pierre, Senior Director of Operations
Lauren McLeod, Editorial Director	

Advice given is general. Readers should consult professional counsel for specific legal, ethical, or clinical questions.

Arrangements can be made for quantity discounts. For more information, contact:

HCPro, Inc.
75 Sylvan Street, Suite A-101
Danvers, MA 01923
Telephone: 800-650-6787 or 781-639-1872
Fax: 800-639-8511
Email: *customerservice@hcpro.com*

Visit HCPro online at *www.hcpro.com* and *www.hcmarketplace.com*

Contents

Contents

Communication 81

Nurturing the Professional Growth of the NPD Specialist 93

Administrative Issues 117

Contents

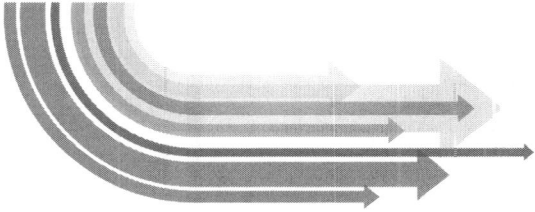

About the Authors

Adrianne E. Avillion, DEd, RN, is the owner of Avillion's Curriculum Design in York, PA, and specializes in designing continuing education programs for healthcare professionals and freelance medical writing. She is the editor of the e-newsletter *Staff Development Weekly* and is a frequent presenter at various conferences and conventions devoted to continuing education and professional development. She is the author of *Evidence-Based Staff Development: Strategies to Create, Measure, and Refine Your Program*; *A Practical Guide to Staff Development: Evidence-Based Tools and Techniques for Effective Education*; Second Edition; and *The Survival of Staff Development: Measure Outcomes and Demonstrate Value to Establish an Indispensable Department.*

Contributing author **Barbara A. Brunt, MA, MN, RN-BC, NE-BC,** is director of nursing education and staff development for Summa Health System in Akron, OH. Brunt is currently serving a two-year term as president of National Nursing Staff Development Organization. She has held a variety of staff development positions, including education coordinator and director, for the past 30 years. Brunt has presented on a variety of topics both locally and nationally and has published numerous articles, chapters, and books. She is a noted author, including *Competencies for Staff Educators: Tools to Evaluate and Enhance Nursing Professional Development*, published by HCPro.

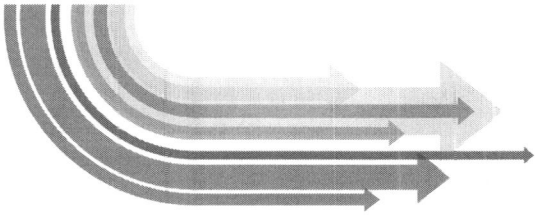

Introduction

Nursing professional development (NPD) specialists occupy a unique position in the healthcare community. We are nurses, educators, change agents, and researchers. We are the "go-to" people when problems arise or encouragement is needed. But to whom do we go when we encounter problems or need encouragement? Most often, the answer is each other.

This book was written to offer NPD colleagues short, relevant bursts of information to help deal with common challenges we encounter in our professional practice. Also provided are a number of resources to consult for more detailed information.

The section on Education and Training provides the reader with tips to successfully cope with the day-to-day challenges of offering education and training to adult learners with a wide range of professional experience. The Communication section is designed to help the NPD specialist remove or reduce barriers to effective communication in healthcare organizations—especially important as research shows that poor communication has an adverse effect on most, if not all, aspects of organizational functioning.

The sections on Nurturing and Professional Growth of NPD Specialist and Administrative Issues are written from the personal perspective of an NPD specialist who wants to help peers design career advancement paths for our specialty as well as add to the unique body of knowledge that is NPD.

It is my hope that readers will use this book as a practical resource to not only effectively overcome common NPD challenges, but to promote the professional growth and development of those whose chosen specialty is nursing professional development.

Adrianne E. Avillion, DEd, RN
Avillion's Curriculum Design
York, PA

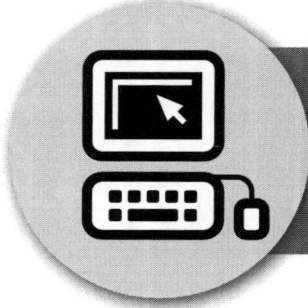

DOWNLOAD YOUR MATERIALS NOW

www.hcpro.com/downloads/10170

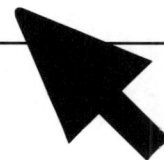

Thank you for purchasing this product!

HCPro

Education and Training

Learning Objectives

- Implement tips for resolving education and training dilemmas.

- Identify the most common challenges regarding education and training.

- Discuss pitfalls when implementing training and education.

Section 1

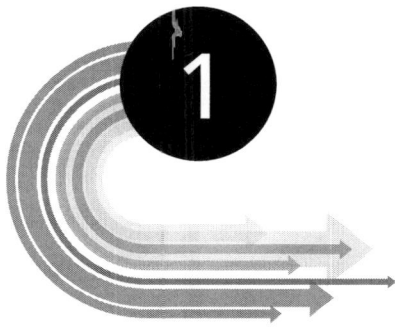

In-service

It's 4:30 p.m. on a Friday afternoon. It's been a hectic week and you're looking forward to the weekend. Just as you begin to think about packing your briefcase and heading for home, your phone rings. It's the charge nurse on one of the oncology units. A patient is being transferred to her unit from another, smaller hospital. The patient has a rare form of cancer and is arriving with some new equipment necessary for treatment with which the staff is unfamiliar. Nor are they very familiar with the particular type of cancer affecting the patient. The charge nurse asks for help educating her staff. New equipment? Unfamiliar diagnosis? Training is needed now! How can we deal more effectively with the need for in-service and on-demand training without allowing this need to turn into another training crisis?

In-service education is often referred to as simple, short-term programming that meets an immediate need (Avillion, 2008). Also referred to as on-the-job or just-in-time training, in-service education often involves the need to master the operation of a new piece of equipment, provide nursing care to a patient with an unfamiliar diagnosis, or implement a new or updated policy or procedure quickly. In other words, in-service education is a rapid response to changes in your work environment (Avillion, 2008).

How can we make responding to the need for in-service education less of a crisis intervention and more of a learning experience? Let's start by dealing with the need to educate staff on new equipment. The first step is to know your vendors.

Know Your Vendors

Maintain a current list of local equipment vendors and/or sales representatives. They are often willing to help with in-services as part of their job responsibilities and generally respond fairly quickly to requests for help. Although they may not be able to come personally, they may be able to transmit training videos online almost immediately. Unfortunately, these people seem to change jobs (and companies) quite often. Assign responsibility for maintaining an up-to-date list to your departmental secretary (if you're fortunate enough to have one) or another member of the department. Sometimes current information can be obtained from a company's website. If not, phone calls need to be made. Updating should be done every month or two but never less frequently than quarterly. If you don't think there is time for someone to do this remember that it takes a lot more time to function in a crisis mode trying to locate your vendors and come up with an in-service on your own. Schedule this "updating" task as you would any other responsibility. In the long run, having a current list of vendors and sales representatives will save you time and energy.

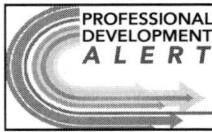

> **PROFESSIONAL DEVELOPMENT ALERT** Suppose you don't have a departmental secretary? In that case contact your director of volunteers. You may be able to acquire the services of a reliable volunteer on a monthly or quarterly basis.

Contact information for vendors should include:

- ❑ Company name and website address

- ❑ What types of equipment they supply

- ❑ Name of your vendors and/or sales representatives

- ❑ What help is available in an emergency situation after regular business hours

- ❑ Phone numbers (both office and mobile phones), e-mail, and preferred method of contact

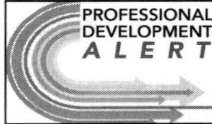

> **PROFESSIONAL DEVELOPMENT ALERT** Find out if the company's website lists the names of local vendors and sales representatives and their contact information. If this is the case, maintaining current information will be a swiftly accomplished task.

Woo your vendors and sales representatives. Include them on your holiday greeting card list. When they help you with in-service education, whether it be in person or by sending education resources, be sure to thank them profusely. Send a follow-up e-mail or text telling them how the education they facilitated helped you and the nursing staff. Offer them coffee when they drop by. Treat them as a friend, not an annoying interruption, no matter how inconvenient the timing. They will be more likely to help someone who treats them with courtesy.

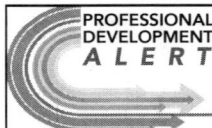

> **PROFESSIONAL DEVELOPMENT ALERT** Encourage nurse managers and clinicians to treat vendors with respect and a welcoming attitude.

Ask your vendors and sales representatives if they have training resources such as DVDs and online in-service videos that can be downloaded to computers, mobile devices, etc. Being able to download these types of teaching tools in a hurry is a big help for you and your learners. Also ask if staff members can access these tools during nonbusiness hours.

Identify Nurses Who Can Help

The next step is to make sure you identify staff nurses who are willing and able to help with in-service. These nurses need to be nurtured and may, someday, be groomed to assume the role of a unit-based educator or nursing professional development (NPD) specialist.

If your organization has a career advancement/clinical ladder program that requires staff to participate in the education of their peers, you can use those requirements to encourage staff nurses to participate in in-service training. Nurses pursuing advancement may be especially willing to learn more about the educator role.

Work with nurse managers to identify nurses who show an interest in and an aptitude for helping to educate others. You are more likely to gain the cooperation of nurse managers by working together and explaining how having their staff nurses trained to help with in-service education is beneficial to all concerned. Don't let nurse managers get the impression that you are trying to take time from their staff members to do your job.

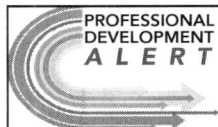

> **PROFESSIONAL DEVELOPMENT ALERT** When working with others to identify staff nurses who are likely candidates to help with in-service, help them to understand that the best clinicians do not necessarily make the best educators. Look for nurses who go out of their way to help educate their colleagues.

If you are fortunate enough to have unit-based educators as part of the professional development department, one of their responsibilities should be to help identify and train staff nurses to help with in-service education. Identifying staff nurses who are interested in helping to educate their peers is one way to identify possible future candidates for the role of unit-based educator.

Offer a train-the-trainer course for identified staff nurses on a regular basis. This is not the same as the preceptor course, although some content may overlap. The train-the-trainer course should focus on in-service, including such issues as the principles of adult learning, dealing with disruptive learners, how to help colleagues who do not meet learning objectives, and resources available for in-service education. Identify staff nurses who are trained to help with in-service on all shifts.

Facilitate a Knowledge Depository

Facilitate a new knowledge "depository" for all units. Arguably, the quickest and easiest source is online. If your department has its own portion of the hospital's intranet, you might develop such a resource. Some units prefer to maintain their own depository, particularly specialty units that have knowledge needs unique to those specialties. The knowledge depository should include:

❑ Access to the organization's online library resources

❑ Software applications (apps)

❑ Other websites (including those of the vendors and sales representatives for critical equipment)

❑ Access to hard copies of relevant journals and books

❑ Contact information for key resources (e.g., vendors, NPD specialists, etc.)

You also need to consider how to document how learners achieve learning objectives. One way to facilitate documentation is to have a template that can be quickly filled out and printed from your computer or, in some documentation systems, complete the form directly on a PDA or other similar devices.

Figure 1.1 (*www.hcpro.com/downloads/10170*) is a sample template for something that requires a review or reading of a document such as a new or revised policy, Joint Commission alerts, etc. The document is something that could be posted either as a hard copy or sent via PDA. Adapt the wording of the template to meet your organization.

Figure 1.2 (*www.hcpro.com/downloads/10170*) is a template that is appropriate for use when a competency, such as safely mastering new equipment or a new procedure, must be demonstrated. Note that there is space for objectives and specific behaviors that must be demonstrated to achieve competency. There is also space to note whether or not competency was achieved and to document necessary remediation if competency is not achieved.

Reference

Avillion, A. E. (2008). *A Practical Guide to Staff Development: Evidence-based Tools and Techniques for Effective Education.* Danvers, MA: HCPro.

2

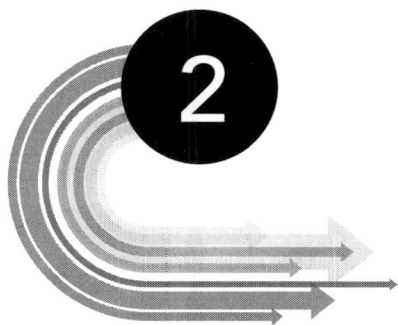

Reviewing and Revising Your Orientation Program

Every nursing professional development (NPD) specialist deals with the ongoing dilemma of orientation. How long should it be? What is too long? What is too short? How can we reconcile learning needs with the needs of the nurse managers who want new nurses ready to assume a full patient assignment sooner rather than later?

Unfortunately there is no single right way to offer orientation. Orientation needs vary according to the size of the organization and the needs of the patient population. As with all NPD activities, any changes in orientation must be grounded in evidence. If your organization uses a shared governance model, you can rely on unit-based councils, leadership councils, quality councils, and the NPD council to work with you on orientation design and revision. If not, you still need to work with persons who would be part of such councils if they existed, such as nurse managers, staff nurses, human resources, quality improvement personnel, and NPD colleagues.

It is not possible to say what should or should not be part of orientation, nor is it possible to identify the correct length of orientation. What is possible is to give you some tips to evaluate and strengthen your orientation program:

- Consider forming a nursing orientation task force or have orientation addressed at least semiannually during unit-based and other councils as part of the shared governance model (if your organization espouses shared governance). The opportunity for members of the nursing staff to have input often helps to control some of the negativity sometimes associated with orientation. It also offers NPD specialists the opportunity to provide evidence (such as turnover rates, rates of competency achievement, etc.) regarding the effectiveness of orientation.

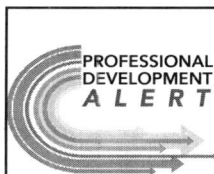

PROFESSIONAL DEVELOPMENT ALERT

Never attend meetings at which orientation will be discussed without your objective evidence. Do not limit yourself to reaction data. You absolutely need to begin (if you haven't already done so) collecting data pertaining to retention and turnover, analyze it, and present your evidential findings. Only by using such evidence will you be able to gain support for orientation and any necessary revisions.

- Meet with preceptors at least semiannually. They are more likely to buy-in to the entire orientation process if they have the opportunity to provide regular input and hear, directly from NPD specialists, the evidence that is available regarding orientation success (or lack of success) and preceptor impact on retention and turnover.

PROFESSIONAL DEVELOPMENT **A L E R T**

> Review the process of preceptor selection. Are all nurses expected to function as preceptors? Is assuming responsibility for preceptorship part of career advancement? Are preceptors compensated for assuming this type of responsibility? One of the major stumbling blocks to an effective preceptor program is to automatically mandate that all nurses function as preceptors. The role of preceptor should be part of a career advancement program and compensated monetarily. Ideally, the preceptor role should be considered both advantageous and prestigious and candidates should apply for the role.

- Implement, review, and revise orientation based on evidence, not complaints or even accolades.

- Orientation will always be a dynamic process, constantly undergoing evaluation and revision. Everyone involved needs to accept this fact. This acceptance makes it easier to accept the idea of frequent change regarding orientation.

- Unit-based orientation varies depending on the experience of the orientee and the rapidity with which she/he learns. Caution preceptors not to expect a newly licensed nurse to complete orientation at the same pace as a nurse with five years of experience. Part of preceptor training should be to never, ever compare new orientees to each other.

PROFESSIONAL DEVELOPMENT **A L E R T**

> Caution preceptors not to assume that an experienced nurse will require less orientation than a newly licensed nurse. Everyone learns at a different pace. The experienced nurse may be entering a new specialty or perhaps has moved from a different geographic location. These types of issues will impact on her/his ability to learn.

- When altering the method of teaching (e.g., going from classroom to computer-based learning [CBL]), be sure to evaluate the change in terms of leaning, behavior, and, whenever possible, results. Compare data prior to the change with data after change is implemented. Doing so allows you to objectively evaluate whether or not the change is beneficial.

- Include information about acquiring a mentor during orientation. Mentors, who do not have supervisory or authority over the orientee, function as part of a support system and career coach. Almost everyone needs a mentor! There are pros and cons to having an in-house mentor. Confidentiality is an important consideration;no new employee wants to discover that his or her concerns and discussions are made public by his or her mentor. It is suggested that mentors do not come from the same unit as the orientee. You may even be able to organize a "mentor exchange" with other organizations and/or colleges and universities with which your organization has student affiliations.

- Include information about bullying during orientation. This should include bullying from supervisory personnel, subordinates, and peers.

PROFESSIONAL DEVELOPMENT ALERT Include information about bullying, especially horizontal bullying (peer against peer), as part of preceptor training. Offer objective data regarding the effectives of bullying and that it is not going to be tolerated.

- Incorporate opportunities for orientation attendees to network after they have moved from general orientation to unit-specific orientation. Some organizations have organized times for orientees to gather periodically throughout their first year of employment. Nurse managers are mandated to release these employees for these meetings. It provides not only a support system but a chance to retrieve valuable data about the orientation process.

In summary, there is no magical solution to orientation because orientation is in a constant state of change. However, by reviewing these suggestions. you will hopefully find ways to deal more effectively with the challenges orientation provides.

3

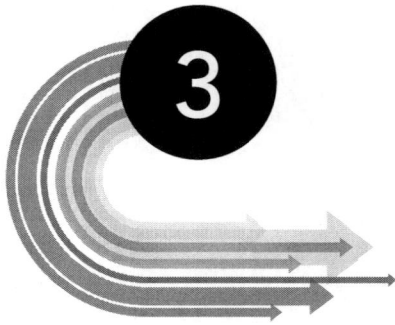

Enhancing Your Preceptor Program

Based on discussions with a number of nursing professional development (NPD) specialists, recurring themes have emerged regarding content and preceptor selection. It is the purpose of this chapter to help you identify some strategies for selecting preceptors and remind you of important content issues.

Preceptor Selection

One of the biggest challenges of NPD is dealing with the way preceptors are identified and selected. In some organizations, although the number is decreasing, all nurses are expected to serve as preceptors. There is no monetary compensation for the extra time it takes to fill the role nor is it part of a career advancement plan (i.e., climbing the clinical ladder). This is *not* a good way to develop a preceptor program. If your organization is still mandating that all nurses serve as preceptors, gather data and provide evidence to prove that this policy should be changed! Most likely,evidence will show that nurses who are not interested in, or who do not have the aptitude for, serving as preceptors will be linked to increased turnover among those new nurses for whom they precept.

When selecting preceptors, keep the following considerations in mind:

- Filling the role of preceptor should be part of a career advancement path. It should not be the only option at a certain step in the path. There are other options for nurses who want to advance in the role of staff nurse (perhaps some have more of an interest in research or managerial duties). Options should and must exist.

- Compensation should be offered for those who serve as preceptors. This compensation may take several forms, such as monetary compensation in hourly wages for those hours they are precepting, additional time off with pay, etc.

- The role of preceptor should be one that is accompanied by prestige and respect. This can only be the case if preceptors earn both.

- Candidates for the role of preceptor should have to apply for the role. They need to be recommended by their nurse managers and possess clinical expertise and an aptitude for educating adults. NPD specialists should also be involved in evaluating candidate applications. Part of the application process should include observing the potential preceptor as she/he provides education such as on-the-job training to peers.

- Implement a support network for preceptors. They need the opportunity to network with each other and with NPD specialists. Arrange for a regular periodic meeting of preceptors. Such meetings will also be a good source of data for NPD specialists and nurse managers as they evaluate the quality of the preceptor program.

- Performance as preceptors must be incorporated as part of their annual job performance evaluation. Evaluation of their effectiveness as preceptors should include objective data that relate to results like retention, turnover, and orientees' successful completion of orientation.

Preceptor Program Content

Some aspects of content will, of course, vary depending on the organization and the specialty of the units involved, but there are some general areas of content that should be included. Based on feedback from NPD colleagues, preceptors should:

- Assess their own learning styles and learn about the learning styles of others. They need to learn how to facilitate learning in preceptees whose learning style is different from their own.

- Perform a confidential self-analysis of their own strengths and weaknesses, such as patience, ability to offer and accept constructive criticism, clinical strengths and weaknesses, etc. They also need to examine their own beliefs and values and how to deal with orientees whose beliefs and values differ from their own.

- Learn principles of adult learning and how to apply them.

- Lean the ethics of functioning as preceptors, including confidentiality.

- Learn legal issues of precepting orientees.

- Recognize the effects of horizontal bullying, including how to recognize bullying behaviors in themselves.

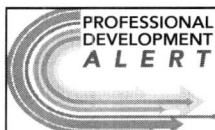

> **PROFESSIONAL DEVELOPMENT ALERT**   Preceptors must also receive training in how to deal with orientees who are bullies. It is less common to have orientees behave in this manner, but it does happen.

- Document orientee performance.

- Identify learning objectives.

- Conduct an objective evaluation of orientees.

- Know how to conclude the preceptor/orientee relationship.

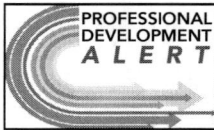

PROFESSIONAL DEVELOPMENT ALERT Incorporate role play as part of the preceptor program. Use challenging simulated situations such as having to tell orientees that they have failed to meet learning objectives, dealing with orientees who are angry and upset, etc.

The preceding issues are guidelines for your own program. There will, of course, be additional content you will wish to provide. The issues described in this chapter are areas that some NPD colleagues have identified as critical to the success of their own preceptor programs.

Nurse Residency Programs

Nurse residency programs are growing in number and popularity. Data in reports such as the Institute of Medicine's *The Future of Nursing* provide evidence that supports healthcare resources efforts to be more fully allotted to recruit, retain, and educate members of the nursing profession. The implementation of nurse residency programs is one way to facilitate the orientation of new nurses and enhance their successful assimilation into an organization so that they can provide the best possible patient care.

If you are thinking of starting a residency program or revising a current program, you need some resources to aid you in your task. There are no regulatory guidelines for such programs, so you have the opportunity to design one that works for the nursing staff and the organization. The ultimate goal of most residency programs is to assist the BSN graduate in his/her transition from student to professional.

The average length of a nurse residency program is about one year, including basic nursing orientation. Benefits vary. For example, some programs provide and pay for specialty preparation courses as well as meetings for the residents to come together to discuss their experiences and network.

A good way to begin working on the development or revision of a residency program is to look at what is already available. A good resource, *Guide to Hospital Nursing Residency Programs for New BSNs*, has been developed by The University of Pennsylvania Career Services (find the document at *www.vpul.upenn.edu/careerservices/nursing/nurseresidency.pdf*). It lists hospitals (and their websites) that provided structured residency programs for new BSNs. Programs are listed alphabetically by state and also identify themselves as to whether they have been designated as an ANCC Magnet Recognition Program® hospital.

Most of the websites contain at least a brief overview of the residency program, including such information as length, some of the content, and programs that are offered for specific specialties. Requirements for eligibility and applications to be accepted into the programs are also available online.

Communicate with other organizations regarding their nurse residency programs. Such communication is probably best with persons whose organizations are at enough of a geographic distance from you so that they won't be afraid of giving information to competitors. Your best resources are probably going to be those who have already been through the trial and error process of developing a nurse residency program.

In discussions with other nursing professional development (NPD) specialists, I have found that some of the biggest challenges occurred as a result of failure to consider and address the following questions. Consider these questions carefully and base your program development on your responses:

- What is administration's response to the concept of a nurse residency program? Will they provide the human and monetary resources necessary for program development and maintenance? Have you provided them with a budget? Have they agreed to that budget?

- What is nursing leadership's response to the concept of a nurse residency program? Do they comprehend the time and resources necessary for its successful implementation? How have the logistics of the program been presented to them? What opportunities have they had to participate in its development?

- Do staff nurses support the concept of a nurse residency program? Have they been involved in its development? Do they understand the roles they will play in the success (or failure) of such a program?

- Who is officially responsible for the nurse residency program? Do the responsible person(s) also have the authority necessary to oversee and supervise the program?

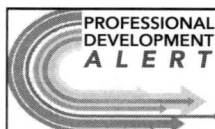

> **PROFESSIONAL DEVELOPMENT ALERT**
>
> Don't accept the responsibility for the nurse residency program unless you also have the authority to effectively manage the program. Responsibility without authority is doomed to failure.

- Who has control over the budget of the nurse residency program? Whoever controls the money has, ultimately, the authority as well.

- Who makes the decisions as to which candidates will be accepted into the nurse residency program? The decisions should be made not only by nurse mangers but in conjunction with their staff members and NPD specialists (if they are involved in program planning, implementation, and evaluation).

- How have you differentiated between orientation and a nurse residency program? Some people may believe that a nurse residency program is just a longer orientation. They need to know that a residency program has specific content and objectives and lasts for a specified length of time.

- How have you assessed the needs of nurses who will enter the nurse residency program? Have you interviewed nurses who have gone through your orientation program but did not have the opportunity to participate in a nurse residency program? Have you talked to nurses who have been through such a program for constructive feedback?

- How has the nurse residency program been planned? What are its objectives? Have representatives from administration, nursing leadership, and staff nurses been involved?

- Who are the people responsible for implementing the program? What education has been provided to those responsible—administration, nursing leadership, and staff nurses—regarding the nurse residency program?

- How will the nurse residency program be evaluated? How often will it be revised? How long has funding been provided for the program?

- Are criteria for acceptance into the program objective and measurable? How will candidates be notified of their acceptance or failure to be accepted?

- Who is responsible for posting criteria on the organization's website? Who will monitor its ongoing accuracy?

Hopefully, addressing these questions in advance will help you in the development of your own nurse residency program.

5

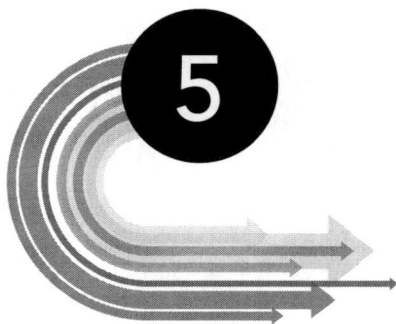

Cultural Diversity Training

Cultural diversity training is continually expanding as the number of cultures represented by patient populations and professional colleagues grows. Many organizations include cultural competence as part of annual mandatory training, using role-play, computer-based learning (CBL), or case studies as teaching/learning tools.

Some organizations have tried to become a bit more innovative. One large health system has initiated an approach where professional colleagues representing various cultures and ethnicities play the role of visitors and patients during learning activities and assess healthcare workers' responses to their questions and concerns. The persons playing the various roles do not role-play in their own facilities (although they might be part of the larger health system). Using unfamiliar people can ease along the role-playing, making it a bit more realistic. This same approach could be initiated by using local faculty from nursing schools with which you have affiliations. Cultural issues incorporated into the role-play include:

- ❑ Eye contact

- ❑ Handshake

- ❑ Personal space

- ❑ Dress

- ❑ Business etiquette

- ❑ Response to pain

- ❑ Dietary issues

- ❑ Family spokesperson issues

- ❑ Caring for persons of the opposite sex

- ❑ Facial expressions and gestures

- ❑ Body language

Many of us already have various types of cultural diversity training in place, but are frustrated by the lack of resources to help us expand our knowledge base of new cultures or new aspects of cultures. Here is a list of resources that should prove helpful to you as you expand your diversity training.

Resources

The following is a list of resources to assist you in diversity training:

- American Association for Respiratory Care. (2012). Cultural diversity resources: Tools for healthcare workers. Retrieved February 19, 2012, from *www.aarc.org/resources/cultural_diversity/tools.cfm*.

- Galanti, G. (2012). Cultural diversity in healthcare. Retrieved February 18, 2012, from *www.gagalanti.com*.

- Hepburn-Smith, M., & Whitmer, K. (2005). Seeking cultural competence. *ADVANCE for Nurses, Pennsylvania, New Jersey, and Delaware*, November 14, 2005, 21-21.

- IAPCC-Rc. (2011). Inventory for assessing the process of cultural competence among healthcare professionals-revised (AIPCC-Rc). Retrieved February 18, 2012, from *www.transculturalcare.net/iapcc-r.htm*.

- James, E. (2005). Ethno-experts. *ADVANCE for Nurses, Pennsylvania, New Jersey, and Delaware*, June 27, 2005, 29-34.

- Pagana, K. D. (2011). Mind your manners multi-culturally. Nurse.com, June 13, 2011, 48-53.

- Taylor, R. (2005). Addressing barriers to cultural competence. *Journal for Nurses in Staff Development*, July/August, 135-144.

- Transcultural Nursing. (2012). Diversity in health and illness. Retrieved February 18, 2012, from *www.culturediversity.org*.

6

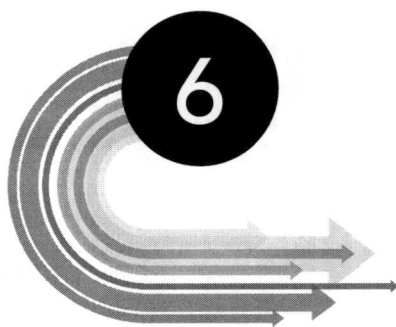

Facilitating the Use of Clinical Evidence-Based Practice

Evidence-based practice (EBP) in the clinical setting is expected and has been adapted in most organizations. Nursing professional development (NPD) specialists are often called upon to facilitate and teach concepts of EBP in the clinical setting.

As in our own NPD EBP, clinicians must apply evidence of best practices to their patient care. How can we facilitate EBP in the clinical settings?

First, we need to determine a system for disseminating research findings that document evidence of best practice. Someone from each unit (ideally a unit-based educator) should assume responsibility for disseminating such information. Information can be obtained with the help of the NPD department, unit-based councils, and education councils. Using the organization's employee portion of its website is an ideal way to direct nurses to journal articles and new findings. If you don't have this option, use bulletin boards, e-mail, or whatever method works best for you. Specific time should be allotted during every staff meeting to discuss best practice evidence, how this evidence can be used, and what research questions are being triggered by this evidence. If your organization has a nurse researcher(s), include them in the process of disseminating information and identifying research questions.

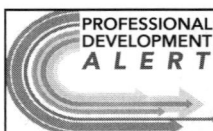

> **PROFESSIONAL DEVELOPMENT ALERT**
> Another excellent resource for EBP is your local Sigma Theta Tau chapter as well as the faculty from your student affiliations. Some faculty collaborate with staff nurses and students to identify research questions and to evaluate best practice evidence.

However, it's not enough to simply disseminate information. Staff nurses need to feel that their professional input matters. They should be involved in identifying their own best practices as they provide patient care. They should also question current policies and procedures if they observe that current practice needs revision based on patient outcomes and literature review.

Steps to facilitate EBP at the bedside should include:

- ❑ Identify a system for disseminating best practice findings and literature reviews.

- ❑ Identify experts such as nurse researchers and clinical faculty who are able to collaborate with nurse leaders and staff nurses to identify best practices and apply them to practice.

- ❑ Incorporate EBP in educational offerings whenever possible.

- ❑ Establish a process for sharing EBP findings, such as at staff meetings, via PDA, etc.

- ❑ Establish a system that allows staff nurses to relay their own opinions and questions about current practice and propose ideas to determine EBP in their own work setting using evidence and research findings as a foundation.

- ❑ Include EBP as part of orientation.

- ❑ Collaborate with university faculty and local chapters of Sigma Theta Tau to enhance EBP education.

One of the best innovations for EBP is the collaboration aspect. Most staff nurses are now accustomed to at least the concept of EBP. The next level of EBP is to promote research into best practices within your own organization, conduct research, and, ultimately, publish and/or present those findings. Remember that the key players in this endeavor are the staff nurses. They should be the key players in any EBP best practice initiatives.

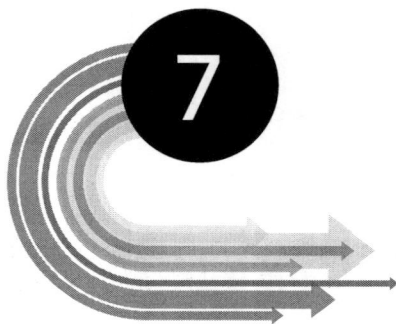

7 Facilitating Competency Assessment

One of the biggest problems with some systems of competency assessment is the large number of checklists and endless reams of paper used to document multitudes of competencies. The competency mandate was never meant to start an avalanche of paper; the mandate was designed to develop a system of ensuring that nurses are competent in their roles and responsibilities. For example, establishing a checklist and monitoring of critical cardiac care nurses' ability to interpret rhythm strips, a task they perform numerous times per shift, is redundant and borders on the ridiculous. How can we simplify the competency assessment process?

First, review orientation competencies. These should be limited to what the orientee must accomplish within the orientation period. These are basic competencies that vary according to the unit and the specialty. Streamline orientation competencies to include only those that are mandatory for completing orientation.

Review the competencies associated with mandatory training. These are mandated by regulatory bodies and organizational standards. Keep these to a minimum as well. For example, what must be demonstrated to be deemed competent in hospital safety according to organizational standards? Correctly use a fire extinguisher? Report a fire? Demonstrate ability to evacuate patients in the event of a fire or other emergency? Review competencies associated with mandatory training annually. Instead of adding more, think about what is truly necessary.

Unit-based competencies must be reviewed at the unit-based level. Nursing professional development (NPD) specialists are facilitators, not the determiners of what competencies are necessary. Staff nurses and their managers must evaluate their practice and decide which behaviors are high risk/high volume and/or high risk/low volume. If actions are so routine that they are performed many times a day, it is doubtful—unless they are extremely high risk—that such actions need to be evaluated as a competency on an annual basis.

Identify ways to document competency without the burden of checklists. For example, suppose all RNs must be deemed competent in starting IVs. For those RNs who perform this task numerous times a week, as in the emergency department, it is not necessary to have a separate checklist for this competency or have the competency monitored by a superior. The standard in the emergency department might simply state that successful initiation of

IV therapy a specific number of times demonstrates competency. For nurses who do not have a frequent opportunity to start IVs, a more formal observation to determine competency might be necessary.

Keep competency at the unit level. NPD specialists should not be responsible for monitoring all nurses' competency. We need to help facilitate and simplify, but not assume responsibility for activities that are truly unit-based. As more and more organizations adopt the shared governance model, unit-based assumption of responsibility for issues such as competency assessment is becoming the norm, not the exception.

Avoid adding competencies unless they are truly necessary. It is tempting to add competencies, the rationale being it is better to have too much competency documentation rather than too little. This is not true!

Competency assessment should be designed to provide evidence that nurses deliver quality and appropriate care. The system should be designed to incorporate a variety of ways to deem competence, such as number of times a behavior is successfully performed. Not all competencies must involve return demonstration and observation. Consider how competency can be measured most simply.

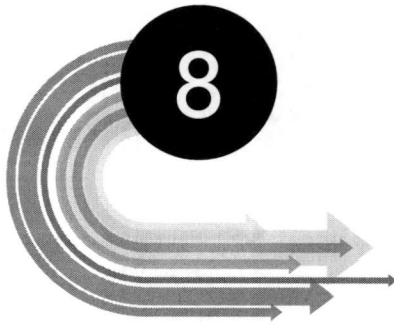

8 Evaluating the Effectiveness of Mandatory Training

Annual mandatory training can take a variety of formats. A significant portion of the training is often available via various computer-based programs. Many organizations have adopted this approach so that learners can access the training at their own convenience. However, some have found that some aspects of mandatory training are viewed as so routine that employees put off accessing the training. Some organizations still incorporate day-long mandatory training events, with classroom, skill demonstration, and computer-based training available. Stations are set up and learners can visit various stations and either access learning at computers, demonstrate psychomotor skills, etc. The important thing is to establish a system that works for your organization and your learners. Most organizations have found that a combination of various formats works best. This approach allows for some flexibility while still allowing for specific skill demonstrations.

When evaluating mandatory training, you need to rely on evidence to measure its effectiveness. Here are some considerations for evaluating the effectiveness of mandatory training:

- Have you identified learning objectives for all facets of the mandatory training? How are you evaluating achievement of these learning objectives? What competencies are associated with these objectives?

- What do the reaction data tell you about mandatory training? What are the comments about format? What do the learners say about the learning environment? How does learner satisfaction affect knowledge acquisition and behavior?

- What mechanisms are in place to measure knowledge? Are you using post-tests? Skills demonstration? Role-play? Is learner satisfaction/dissatisfaction having an impact on learning? What does learner satisfaction tell you about the need to revise the format or the assessment of learning?

- What behaviors are observed in the actual work setting that reflect learning during mandatory training? For example, are learners better able to demonstrate competency during emergency training drills after participating in safety training? Is there evidence of decreased patient complaints or decreased turnover after annual communication skills review? You need to establish a mechanism, preferably unit-based, to monitor behaviors that reflect the effectiveness of mandatory training.

- What are the results of mandatory training? Statistics, such as percentage of employees who attend training (hopefully, 100%), are important, especially because accrediting organizations will ask about this. But far more important are data indicating mandatory training has an actual impact on job performance and patient outcomes. For example, some organizations include some aspects of clinical training during annual mandatory training, especially if the organization is recognized as having specific credentials, such as a designated trauma center or stroke center. In cases such as these, decreased lengths of stay, improved patient outcomes, etc., can be linked to mandatory training.

- Return on investment is a bit more problematic. You may be able to link some types of mandatory training into dollars and cents. The more evidence that demonstrates a link between mandatory training and positive patient outcomes and job performance you can acquire, the better. Such evidence must be shared with employees who make time and take effort to participate in mandatory training. They need to know that it is not just an exercise to satisfy Joint Commission requirements. The reason for participation is to improve both job performance and patient outcomes.

Remember that mandatory training must be evaluated in terms of impact on job performance and/or patient outcomes. At the very least, an increase in knowledge should be demonstrated.

9

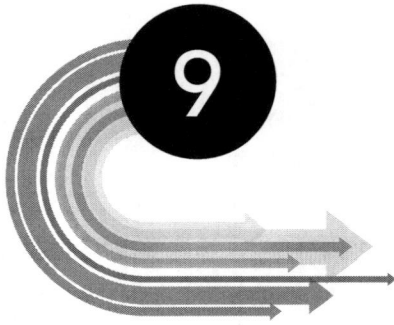

Developing and Maintaining Mentorship Programs

Research shows that mentorships enhance job satisfaction and increase retention. However, some organizations still make no distinction between a mentor and a preceptor. What a mistake! Let's start by differentiating between the two roles.

Preceptors have a limited, time-fixed relationship with orientees. The role of the preceptor is to facilitate the orientee's assimilation into the organization and achieve the competencies necessary to successfully complete orientation. Preceptors have authority over the orientee and supervisory responsibilities. Preceptors evaluate the orientee and have significant input into whether or not the orientee completes orientation (Avillion, 2011).

Mentors function as support systems and career coaches. Theirs is a supportive relationship that has no fixed length of time. Mentors have no authority over those that they mentor. Mentors are experienced practitioners who serve as role models and help mentees to identify and achieve their own career goals (Avillion, 2011).

When starting or evaluating a mentor program, it is important to ask potential mentors the following questions:

❑ Do you have the patience to mentor someone who is new to nursing?

❑ Do you have the time and interest to serve as a mentor? Mentors are almost always voluntary roles and seldom receive monetary compensation unless your organization chooses to do so.

❑ Do you have the experience appropriate to serve as a role model for those you want to mentor?

❑ Might you feel threatened by new employees or colleagues who are enthusiastic and may even eventually compete with their mentors in a chosen specialty?

There are positives and negatives to having a mentor program that matches mentors and mentees who work in the same organization. Positive aspects of such a match include:

• The mentor will understand the culture of the organization, its strengths, and its weaknesses, and its political pitfalls.

- The mentor can help the mentee navigate through the organizational culture and apply for career advancement.

- Working within the same organization may make it easier for both to find time to meet.

Negative aspects of mentoring someone within the same organization include (Avillion, 2011):

- The mentor will not bring fresh perspectives, but instead will approach mentoring from the same organizational cultural perspectives.

- Confidentiality is a concern. The mentee may be fearful that confidential discussions can be overheard or that the mentor may unwittingly share information that the mentee prefer be kept between the two of them.

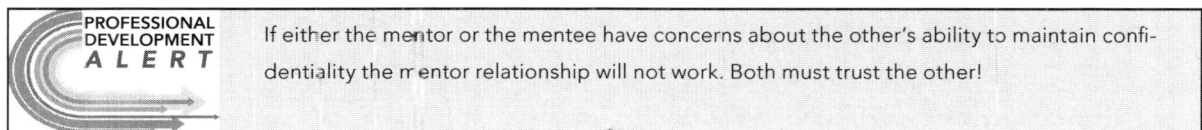

> **PROFESSIONAL DEVELOPMENT ALERT**
>
> If either the mentor or the mentee have concerns about the other's ability to maintain confidentiality the mentor relationship will not work. Both must trust the other!

A mentor from outside the organization brings a new perspective and is not ingrained in the "same old ways of doing things." He or she is also less likely to become involved in any breach of confidentiality, however unwittingly. However, depending on the geographic distance between them, getting together may be more problematic than if they worked in the same organization.

Some people prefer to have a bit of geographic distance between them. In our virtual world, we can meet not only via telephone but via computer and chat and see each other online. Remember that mentors can be hundreds, even thousands of miles away!

When helping to set up a mentor program, you can start by identifying those who want to be mentors. They can be persons from within and outside the organization. The important thing to remember when establishing a mentor program is to identify those people who truly *want* to be mentors and have the time and knowledge necessary to nurture their colleagues.

Mentor programs can be formal or informal. You can make it as simple as maintaining a list of mentors and/or resources for mentors from within or outside the organization. Or you can establish a more formal system.

If you are establishing a mentor program within your organization, you need to offer some education about the mentor role. Education would include:

- ❑ Differentiation between a mentor and a preceptor.

- ❑ Characteristics of a good mentor.

- ❑ Self-evaluation of mentor candidates (see questions at the beginning of this chapter).

- ❑ The roles mentors can play: performance coach, support system, role model.

- ❑ Setting limits: Mentors should be available to their mentees, but within certain parameters.

- ❑ The importance of confidentiality.

- ❑ How to end a mentor relationship.

- ❑ Identifying desired characteristics of mentees: Not all mentors want to fill the role, for example, of a brand new graduate. They may prefer to mentor a nurse who has some experience and is entering a new phase of her/his career or entering a new specialty.

- ❑ How many people is the mentor willing to mentor at one time?

Establish written guidelines based on the education provided and maintain a list of persons who are willing to serve as mentors.

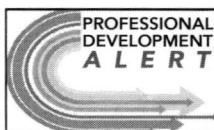

> **PROFESSIONAL DEVELOPMENT ALERT** Make it clear that you are not responsible for "making" a mentor/mentee relationship work. That is the responsibility of the persons involved in the mentor relationship.

You should also have resources available to guide persons to mentors outside the organization. Such resources would include:

- ❑ Local colleges and universities

- ❑ Local and national chapters of professional associations. (Associations often maintain a list of persons who are willing to serve as mentors. Encourage persons looking for a mentor to join professional associations. They might be able to identify their own mentor.)

- ❑ Websites of professional associations, colleges and universities, nurse entrepreneurs, etc. This may give some ideas about persons who are well-known in nursing and contact information.

❑ Local, regional, and national education programs, conferences, and conventions. These are great places to network.

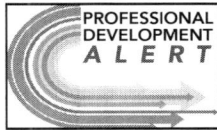

PROFESSIONAL DEVELOPMENT **ALERT**	Never assume responsibility for finding a mentor for someone. This puts you in the position of making the relationship "work." You are providing suggestions to reliable resources, not establishing the relationship.

Don't forget about the need for a mentor for yourself. People assume that only nurses new to the profession need mentors. We all need someone to serve as a sounding board, support system, and guide.

Reference

Avillion, A. E. (2011). *Professional Growth in Staff Development: Strategies for New and Experienced Educators.* Danvers, MA: HCPro.

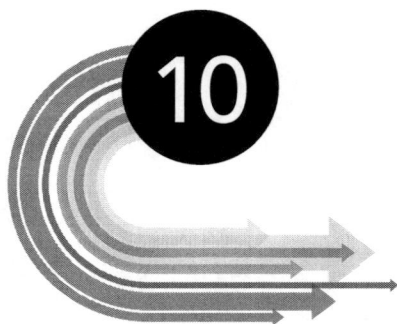

10 Conducting Needs Assessments

Conducting needs assessments can be a frustrating experience. At one time or another most nursing professional development (NPD) specialists have been buried under a mountain of data that is disorganized and fails to help them effectively prioritize and plan education. How can we simplify the needs assessment process?

Obviously we need to gather data regarding educational needs. However, we need to do it as efficiently as possible. Traditionally, many NPD departments conduct an annual needs assessment survey in addition to gathering data from many sources. If an annual survey helps you to gather data and it works for you, then continue to do so! But many such annual surveys are conducted only to satisfy a Joint Commission or other accrediting body requirement. Don't waste time and effort if you only get a minimum number of responses that fail to provide you with useful data. Accrediting bodies are looking for evidence that you are assessing needs, that learners are involved in identifying needs, and that needs are in alignment with organizational goals and priorities. Therefore, an annual survey is not necessary unless it truly provides data that is useful. Figure 10.1 (*www.hcpro.com/downloads/10170*) is an example of a needs assessment form that can be used as an annual survey or at other times. Note that it asks the learner to specifically identify education needs that would help enhance job performance.

You need to evaluate your system of data retrieval and how it is organized. Here are some tips for organizing the needs assessment data collection process:

- Establish or refine your computerized system of documenting and monitoring needs assessment data. There are a number of education tracking systems on the market. Work with your information systems department to select the one that best meets your needs, or work with them to design your own system to track needs assessment data.

- Decide how you will organize the data into education categories. What types of categories will work best for you? Don't get too specific or you will end up repeating the same or similar topics in a number of categories. Categories that are rather broad—pathophysiology, physical assessment, communications, etc.—allow you to put specific items under each. For example, suppose you receive a number of requests for programs on physical assessment, but specific body systems are mentioned. These specifics can be listed under the physical assessment category. There will always be some questions as to what need belongs with which category; however, the more comfortable you get with identifying categories and refining your system, the easier it will be.

- Identify and document your sources of data collection. These would include learners, management, leadership council, quality council, etc. You need to know where your data come from. When organizing your data, you should include its source along with the need.

- Establish a system for reviewing data on a regular basis. Although you can't collect needs assessment data at every committee meeting that occurs, if you establish a semiannual or quarterly time frame, you will keep on top of the data coming in and allow yourself time to organize it.

- Prioritize data according to organizational goals, objectives and areas that have the potential for significant patient impact.

You also need to think about the sources of data. There is so much data available that it can be easy to become overwhelmed. One way to avoid this is for NPD department members to sit down and specifically identify where and how you are collecting data. Consider the following sources of data:

- **Performance evaluations:** Because of confidentiality, NPD specialists do not have direct access to performance evaluations. You need to establish a system so that nurse managers keep a listing of education needs identified during performance evaluations and send you that information without compromising staff identities.

- **Program evaluations:** These types of data are received on a weekly and sometimes daily basis. The NPD secretary should be trained, if possible, to categorize data from these types of evaluations and document them in the computerized system.

- **Councils/committees:** You should be obtaining data from councils/committees including, but not limited to: quality, leadership, education, unit-based, risk management, and infection control.

- **Special events:** All organizations sponsor special events such as Nurse Week. What kinds of events involve large numbers of employees? Are there specific locations, such as the cafeteria, where employees go to participate in special events? If so, consider setting up a table in these locations and gather data feedback from attendees.

In summary, you need to establish a system for collecting, categorizing, and analyzing needs assessment data on a regular basis. This system should not rely on an annual survey, but on a regular process of collecting and documenting data.

Reference

Avillion, A. E. (2008). *A Practical Guide to Staff Development: Evidence-based Tools and Techniques for Effective Education* (2nd ed.). Danvers, MA: HCPro.

The Path to Stress-Free Nursing Professional Development

11 Considering a Distance Learning Format

It wasn't too long ago that the phrase *distance learning* was new and somewhat controversial. Today, it is often the norm. Many nursing professional development (NPD) specialists are caught up in a new dilemma: when is it appropriate to change from a classroom or blended learning format to an all-distance format? This proposed change may be the result of a request from managers that nurses spend less time away from the unit, an administrative request to find less expensive ways of providing education, or the NPD department's belief that a distance format is more cost-effective and learner-friendly.

All of these are reasonable requests. But, before you make a change in format, look at the evidence you have to support or negate such a change. Analyze any proposed change by:

- Examining the reasons for the proposed change. Are these reasons justifiable?

- Asking yourself: What evidence exists for the program's effectiveness in its current format? What types of evaluation have been conducted (e.g., reaction, learning, behavior, results)?

- Piloting the program in a distance learning format before making a permanent change. By piloting the program you can compare evaluation data and determine if a distance format is as effective, less effective, or more effective than the original format.

- Implementing change based on evidence. If the distance format results in improved job performance, then distance is probably the way to go. If the results are poor, then you will have evidence to support a decision not to change the format. However, if the outcomes of both formats are the same, you need to look at time and cost-effectiveness as variables that will help you make your decision.

Whenever you are considering a change, always rely on your evidence-based practice data. By relying on evidence you will have objective data to justify any changes (or lack of changes) you decide to make.

© 2012 HCPro, Inc.

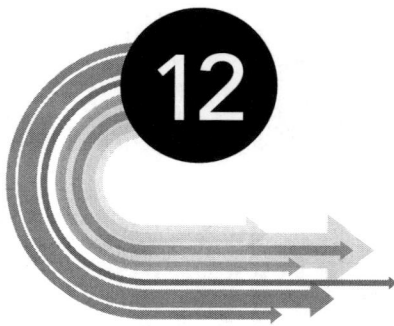

12 Developing an Effective Education Council

As organizations move swiftly to a shared governance model, the importance of an education council cannot be overemphasized. The purpose of an education council is to identify learning needs, facilitate the implementation of education, and evaluate effectiveness of the education provided. Some councils are strictly nursing councils, while others may involve the entire organization. That determination is based on the size and scope of the organization. For example, a large health system with a huge nursing department may limit its role to dealing with the in-service and continuing education of members of the nursing department. A small facility may benefit from having a council that is interdisciplinary in nature. There is no one correct way of developing an education council.

A nursing council allows for focus on nursing and its needs. An interdisciplinary council has the advantage of fostering interdisciplinary teamwork and enhancing patient outcomes by bringing a variety of patient care providers together. Some organizations have both a nursing education council and an education council that is interdisciplinary. Before deciding which option is best for you, find out what support exists for each option. Ask yourself, what format would work best for developing the most effective education in your organization?

The ideal size of a council is between seven and 15 members and length of service is generally two years. Terms should be created so that only half the council is new at any one time (Swihart, 2011). For example, as half of the members begin their first year of service, the other half will be beginning their second year of service. This necessitates that when the council is first established, some members will need to serve either one or three-year terms.

Identifying members can be a challenge. Ideally, they should be volunteers who have a real interest in promoting education that has a positive impact on job performance and patient outcomes. Some organizations have staff nurses submit their names to their unit-based councils and are appointed by that council. Other organizations have their nurse managers appoint members. You may need to try several options for selection until you find the one that is right for your organization. Avoid having the same members serve repetitively. It might be wise to mandate that a nurse who completes his or her two-year term cannot serve again for at least another two years. This gives other nurses the opportunity to serve on the education council.

All education council members deserve an orientation to the education process and how data are collected to evaluate education programs. Most staff nurses are not familiar with the five levels of program evaluation (reaction, learning, behavior, results/impact, and return on investment). Educate staff nurses about these levels and how data are collected for each.

After determining the type of councils needed (i.e., nursing education or interdisciplinary education). you need to clarify your decision by establishing goals and objectives for the council. Obviously, the goals are to design education that improves both job performance and patient outcomes. But what objectives will help to achieve this goal? The council should develop and prioritize objectives and goals based on needs assessment data and organizational priorities.

Here are some questions to consider as you continue to develop your education council.

- Will the education council be strictly a nursing council or will it be an interdisciplinary council? A nursing council allows for focus on nursing and its needs. An interdisciplinary council has the advantage of fostering interdisciplinary teamwork and enhancing patient outcomes by bringing a variety of patient care providers together. Some organizations have both a nursing education council and an education council that is interdisciplinary.

- What will be the format of the council meetings? For example, will there be all-day meetings on a quarterly basis? Half-day meetings bi-monthly?

- How will information regarding education needs be shared? What is the format for presenting needs assessment data?

- How will you share evidence regarding the effectiveness of education? It is imperative that council members be kept apprised of objective evidence and be involved in the review and revision of education efforts.

- Are there particular programs that deserve special attention? Orientation and preceptor training are programs that have a huge impact on the nursing department. Identify other programs for which you particularly need input and support.

- How will you disseminate the information from the education council to other members of the nursing department or interdisciplinary team depending on the nature of the council or council(s)? Make sure any communication coming from the education council is grounded in evidence-based practice.

- What policies and/or guidelines will you need to run an effective education council? For example, do you want a philosophy that mentions confidentiality, that the opinions of all members are respected, etc.? It is best to have "ground rules" developed by the council and respected by all members.

The answers to the preceding questions are important whether you have an established council or are in the process of evaluating your current structure. Remember that the education council will be held accountable, in large part, for the effectiveness of NPD activities.

Reference

Swihart, D. (2011). *Shared Governance: A Practical Approach to Transform Professional Nursing Practice, Second Edition*. Danvers, MA: HCPro, Inc.

13

Simulation as a Teaching Strategy

When you hear the word "simulation" in relation to education and training, many people immediately envision sophisticated equipment like mannequins that breathe, die, and realistically simulate problems such as cardiac arrhythmias. However, not all organizations have the financial resources for such equipment. Even if such equipment is available, there is more to simulation than expensive equipment.

According to the Society for Simulation in Healthcare (*https://ssih.org*) simulation education is a bridge between classroom learning and real-life experience in the actual work setting. Sophisticated equipment is certainly a fabulous option and an invaluable one. However, there are a number of ways to use simulation in addition to this type of equipment. The following are some creative simulation ideas.

Standardized Patients as Part of Simulation

Standardized patients (SP) are individuals trained to portray characters such as patients, families, physicians, nurses, etc., in a simulated patient scenario. They have been in use in medical schools since the 1960s. SPs are given information about a healthcare scenario and how to behave in the simulated scenario. They are also part of the debriefing after the simulation to provide feedback and observations (Amick, B. 2010; Kisner, T., & Johnson-Anderson, H. 2010; Klipfel, J., et al, 2011; Quality and Safety in Education for Nurses, 2011). A good resource for information about SPs is the website of the Association of SP Educators: *www.aspeducators.org*. This organization is the national association for individuals who recruit and train SPs for simulation experience.

Using SPs is an additional expense. These are trained professionals who expect to be financially compensated for their work. However, there are often staff members and nursing professional development (NPD) department members who are able and willing to role-play various scenarios.

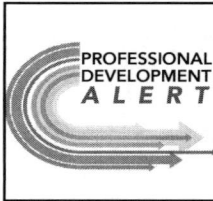

> **PROFESSIONAL DEVELOPMENT ALERT**
>
> If you want to initiate mock emergency drills, mock Joint Commission surveys, etc., you may find that using staff members takes away some of the realism of the situation because they are known to the persons who are participating in the education experience. You may want to collaborate with colleagues from other organizations or the nursing departments of local colleges and ask them to assume the roles of patients, visitors, etc.

Interactive Theater

Similar in some ways to the use of standardized patients, interactive theater is a technique that has learners participate in skits designed to place them in simulated situations of varying degrees of complexity and stress. This technique can be especially helpful when working on communication skills, dealing with horizontal violence, and learning to defuse potentially volatile situations such as angry patients or visitors.

Trained actors, such as SPs, or talented staff members or NPD specialists act out scripted scenarios. Learners enter into the scenario at any point to improve the situation (Meng, A. L., & Sullivan, J. 2011).

Cost-Effective Props

Almost all simulation techniques involve role play or simulated practice of various psychomotor or psychosocial techniques. There are a number of ways to simulate items such as blood, burns, or jaundice using things that you find in any home or local community theaters. For example,

- **Blood:** One bottle of Karo® corn syrup, two bottles of red food coloring, and a few drops of blue food coloring. Mix well and apply to injured "patients."

- **Bruising:** Crumble and mix old blue and green eye shadows into a powder and apply to skin with a soft brush.

- **Burns:** One bottle of theatrical "liquid latex," one bottle of glycerin, and one tube of theatrical grease paint in black. Paint on and smooth out liquid latex over the person or mannequin as a thin film and allow to dry. Be sure that your actor is not allergic to latex before you apply it! When dry, pinch up portions of the film to simulate the appearance of burn blisters.

- **Jaundice:** Wrap the face of a mannequin with yellow plastic wrap. Do *not* use this technique on real people!

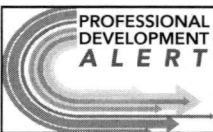

> **PROFESSIONAL DEVELOPMENT ALERT**
>
> Consider making simulation "recipes" a contest for staff members. Ask them to come up with the most realistic simulations using items found in the home. It's a fun idea and gets some buy-in from the staff.

References

Amick, B. (2010). Simulations moulage. Retrieved November 17, 2010, from *www.inquiry.net/outdoor/skills/instruction/simulations.htm.*

Kisner, T., & Johnson-Anderson, H. (2010). Simulation on a shoestring budget. *Nursing,* 40(8), 32-36.

Klipfel, J., et al (2011). Using high-fidelity simulation to develop nurse-physician teams. *The Journal of Continuing Education in Nursing,* 4,2(8), 347-357.

Meng, A. L., & Sullivan, J. (2011). Interactive theater *Journal for Nurses in Staff Development,* 27(2), 65-68.

Quality and Safety in Education for Nurses (QSEN). Simulation exercises. Retrieved March 2, 2012, from *www.qsen.org/search. php?id=19&text=.*

Society for Simulation in Healthcare (SSH). *https://ssih.org.*

14

Making Use of the Unit-Based Educator

Description of the unit-based educator or advanced beginner in the nursing professional development (NPD) arena is described in the Administrative and Nurturing Professional Growth sections of this book. In summary, the role is that of an assistant to the NPD specialist. The unit-based educator's qualifications do not include a graduate degree unless you have determined that particular units require the services of an NPD specialist. More often, the unit-based educator (UBE) focuses on in-service development and implementation, particularly on just-in-time training. How can you best use, and justify, this role? Here are some tips:

- Identify how the UBE will impact job performance at the unit level. Will in-services be more frequent, more timely, or have a more positive impact on job performance and patient care?

- Identify how the UBE will assist the NPD specialist. Ideally, the UBE will be instrumental in helping to conduct needs assessments, implementing in-service, and helping the NPD specialist to evaluate the effectiveness of education.

- Link UBE services to evidence-based NPD practice. Document how the assistance of the UBE allows the NPD specialist more time to implement more advanced levels of practice (e.g., NPD research, evaluating results and return on investment, etc.) and why this is important to organizational effectiveness.

- Link the role of the UBE to education services around-the-clock. Some organizations hire UBEs to work strictly on evening and night shifts and on weekends. This enhances education delivery. Be sure to document evidence as to how such staffing affects job performance and patient care.

- Identify UBEs who are seeking to advance to the role of the NPD specialist. Facilitate the UBE's progress on a career advancement path.

- Use the UBE role to help evaluate preceptor effectiveness and unit-based orientation. Link the role to positive retention outcomes.

- Use the UBE role to enhance relations between NPD specialists, nurse managers, and staff nurses.

- Ensure that UBEs are made to feel a part of the NPD department. Because they spend so much of their time on particular unit(s), they may feel more of an allegiance to the unit than to the NPD department. They are first and foremost, members of the NPD department.

The preceding tips should help trigger some thoughts about how to increase the effectiveness of the UBE role. In turn, the NPD specialist can help the UBE advance professionally and pursue the role of NPD specialist.

15

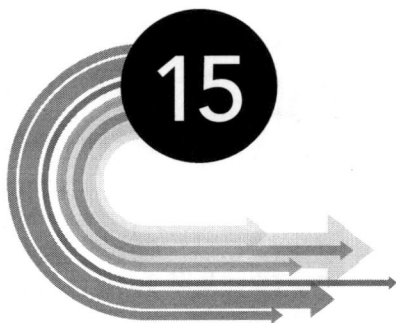

Reducing the Risk of Common Errors

Falls and medication errors seem to be a common source of concern and dismay among all healthcare professionals. Nursing professional development (NPD) specialists are often called upon to come up with education strategies to help reduce the incidence of these and other errors. These kinds of requests often create a dilemma. Do errors occur as a result of a lack of knowledge or a systems issue? We need to be cognizant of strategies to deal with requests for instant remediation. But what strategies can we implement to provide ongoing education about preventing errors?

First of all we need to avoid the typical approach of reviewing the eight rights of medication administration or listing safety measures like making sure the call light is within reach of patients to avoid falls. I don't mean to say that these things are bad, but nurses will either be bored or insulted by such commonplace approaches.

We need to think creatively. How about visual illustrations? Draw a picture of a patient area with about 10 to 15 safety violations and post it wherever learners are most likely to see it (e.g., bulletin boards, computer screens, hospital newsletter, etc.). Offer a prize (e.g., free lunch or dinner in the cafeteria) for the first 10 nurses, or others as appropriate, who correctly identify the violations. Making a contest with a reward attached generates discussion and stimulates interest.

Similarly, write a scenario involving a medication error. Ask nurses to respond by identifying at what point(s) the error could have been prevented. Include a variety of points, including the order being transcribed incorrectly, mislabeling at the pharmacy, failure to check two patient identifiers, etc. Or ask the nursing staff to come up with a creative scenario about error prevention. Create guidelines and make it a contest with members of the education council or another groups acting as judges.

Beyond the Fun Stuff

The preceding ideas incorporate fun ways to learn, which is particularly important to generation Y nurses. However, errors are certainly serious. Is information about error rates and their impact shared with staff nurses? Do they know the scope of the problem within your organization? Do they know the impact? Sadly, many nurses are only given statistics like the number of medication errors, but not the impact on length of stay, stress on staff, and/or monetary costs. How can we expect nurses to truly become involved in error prevention if they don't know what's going on?

Error prevention makes for a good research project. Staff nurses are the bedside experts and the ones most likely to identify ways to prevent errors. Staff nurses should be members of committees and/or councils like quality, risk management, education, etc., so they can have input into the process of increasing the safety of all who are patients or employees within the organization. Their efforts at identifying research questions pertaining to reduction of errors should be supported and encouraged. Thanks to the expanding influence of shared governance, this is happening more and more.

Offering education beyond the basic facts and involving staff nurses in the process of error prevention is necessary. Incorporating fun as part of a serious topic helps encourage learning and limits feelings of fear and discouragement.

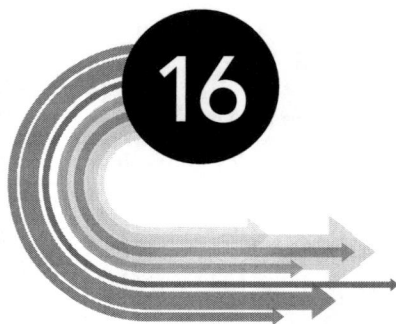

16 Dealing With Disruptive Learners

We've all had to deal with learners who are disruptive. They may be fearful or bored or, in some rare cases, just want to make trouble. Here are some ways to deal with disruptive learners (Avillion, 2008).

First, this is a problem that will always be with us. It is part of the job and we need to be prepared to deal with it. Second, don't blame yourself for an adult's lack of motivation unless the learning activity is truly poorly designed and implemented. Adults are responsible for their own learning. Finally, never ignore disruptive behavior. This will increase it and interfere with the learning experience for everyone who participates.

Motivating Learners

Motivation can seem elusive, but there are strategies you can implement to help increase motivation among your learners. Try the following strategies:

- Explain why this program is being presented. Include learning objectives and rationale.

- Present any evidence you have that the education will have a positive impact on patient outcomes, job performance, and/or organizational effectiveness.

- Explain how evaluation data are to be used. For example, such data will not only help you to improve education offerings, but may help to identify best practices, promote career advancement, etc.

- Identify possible causes of resistance, which may include:

  - **Inappropriate audience:** Have you appropriately identified your audience? Is the program content suitable to the learners' experience?

  - **Teaching strategies:** Have you included a variety of teaching strategies to appeal to different types of learners?

- **Fear:** Are learners afraid of repercussion if knowledge is not acquired? What are these repercussions? Are they real or incorrect assumptions?

- **Credibility:** Are presenters knowledgeable and credible regarding to the topic?

- **Attitude:** Are presenters enthusiastic and supportive of the education and its outcomes?

Identifying motives for lack of motivation can make you a powerful teacher.

Dealing With Overt Hostility

There are many ways to disrupt a learning experience. Asking inappropriate questions, whispering or giggling during a presentation, or monopolizing discussions are a few examples. Here are some ways to defuse the situation:

- Be prepared to insert small group activities or stretch breaks if a learner is causing a disruption. This will draw attention away from him or her. Ask to speak to the person in private during the break. Allowing the disrupter to relay concerns may have a calming effect. Never embarrass the disrupter. This may cause the rest of the learners to support the problem and turn on you.

- If someone continues to disrupt the class don't be afraid to ask him/her to leave the education setting. You cannot allow one or two people to disrupt education for everyone else.

- If the disrupter is asking inappropriate questions, redirect. Explain that those questions are not appropriate for the situation and why they are not. Offer to discuss concerns privately and keep your word to do so.

- If the disrupter is monopolizing a discussion, redirect. Explain that time is limited but offer to meet with him or her later to continue the discussion. This is often enough to defuse the situation.

- Always keep calm no matter how upset or annoyed you are. Anger and frustration are contagious and you will soon have a room full of frustrated adults.

Although you shouldn't react emotionally to disruptive learners, you shouldn't ignore them either. Critically assess why the disruption is occurring and implement strategies to minimize the disruptions.

Dealing With the Potentially Violent Learner

Some learners are so angry that violence is a possibility. For example, if someone fails an exam or fails to achieve competency, his or her job status may be in jeopardy. Remember, when dealing with the possibility of verbal or physical violence:

- Encourage the angry person to sit down. Keep on the same eye level.

- Speak in a calm, measured tone of voice. Never raise your voice or let your voice or body language indicate anger or fear.

- Don't take the person's anger personally. The real source of anger may be someone else such as a manager, spouse, or friend.

- Listen actively. Maintain eye contact, nod your head, and show that you want to help resolve the problematic issues.

- Never allow an angry person to get between you and the exit. Make sure you have easy access to get out of an office or classroom. Don't let yourself be trapped with a potentially violent person.

- Know how to summon help. Don't be afraid to call for help if you are in danger.

- If you suspect a possibility of violence, don't meet with the person alone, or make sure that someone else knows of the potential for trouble and is stationed nearby.

- Report incidents of violence. Never allow violence—threatened or actual—to go unreported. Follow your organization's procedures for reporting such problems.

Violence is unacceptable. Be sure to lean on support whenever needed.

Reference

Avillion, A. E. (2008). *A Practical Guide to Staff Development: Evidence-based Tools and Techniques for Effective Education.* Danvers, MA: HCPro.

The Path to Stress-Free Nursing Professional Development

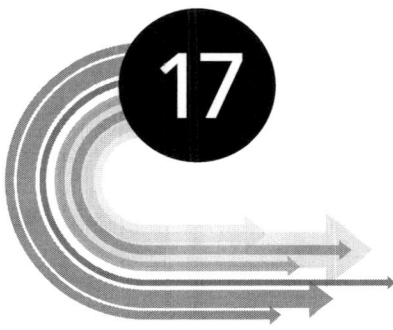

17 Enhancing Your Presentation Skills

Presentation skills are important to all nursing professional development (NPD) specialists. Whether it be presenting mandatory training or presenting a paper at a national conference, these skills need to be polished.

Here are some ideas for enhancing your presentation skills:

- **Be prepared.** This may sound self-evident, but trying to find time to rehearse your presentation is difficult. However, in order to come across as a credible speaker and reduce your own nervousness, you need to be thoroughly familiar with your topic.

- **Be innovative.** This is especially important if you are presenting the same topic(s) over and over ,such as mandatory training or orientation. For your own sake, as well as your learners', change things around a bit. Change the order of topics, add a game, or include more options for discussion.

- **Take breaks.** Incorporate stretch breaks for you and the audience at least once an hour to help everyone stay focused. This is especially important if you are teaching lengthy sessions.

- **Be enthusiastic!** Keep your tone of voice upbeat and look interested in what you are saying and what your learners are saying.

- **Share credentials.** Learners want to know that you have both the credentials and expertise to present on your topic. Limit such information to a few sentences, otherwise it will come across as overbearing.

- **Modulate your tone of voice.** Speak loudly enough to be heard but don't shout. Use a lower pitched tone and avoid high, squeaky tones. Speak at a moderate pace. If you're too quick, you won't be understood; too slow, and you'll put your learners to sleep.

- **Make eye contact.** Make your learners feel that you are speaking directly to them.

- **Smile.** Keep a pleasant expression on your face for a positive and engaging connection with your audience.

- **Don't turn your back on your audience for more than an instant.** You will give the impression of not caring or of being uncertain.

- **Avoid looking at your wristwatch.** Place a watch next to your notes or in a location where you can glance at it and not be obvious.

- **Emphasize objectives.** Make sure learners know what they are going to learn and why.

- **Share evidence.** You are much more likely to trigger interest if learners know that the topic has relevance to their professional life.

- **Don't read your presentation.** You can rely on notes, but don't give the impression of reading to your learners.

- **Make sure your equipment works.** Always check on the status of any equipment *before* you start your presentation.

- **Encourage discussion and learner participation.**

- **Don't let one person monopolize the learning session.** Although you want to encourage discussion, you can't let one person take over. You can always thank them for his or her interest, explain that you must proceed, and offer the option of continuing a discussion with him or her at break or at a later time in your day.

- **Learn from constructive criticism.** Ask a trusted colleague to evaluate your presentation skills from time to time. We all fall into bad habits and sometimes we need help from a trusted, objective source to get us back on track.

Even the most experienced presenter can benefit from an objective analysis of his or her presentation skills. We can all improve—and retain our enthusiasm for presenting—by taking the time to evaluate ourselves (with the help of others).

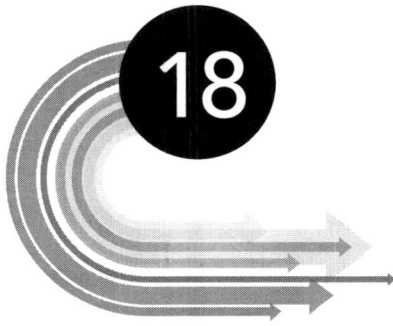

Innovative and Appropriate Teaching Strategies

18

Choosing the appropriate teaching strategy should always be grounded in evidence. What format has the most positive impact on achieving desired results? This is the most important reason for choosing a format and has been discussed in various chapters throughout this book. After addressing the issue of impact, consider cost, time, and ease of accessibility.

Don't just focus on classroom, simulation, and computer-based learning; some "old" tried-and-true methods that may have fallen into disuse thanks to technological advances work well. In fact, some of the older approaches are now considered innovative and provide relief from what can be a bombardment of technology. Here are some ideas:

- **Bulletin boards:** Remember when bulletin boards were essential to communication? They can still be useful. They are usually located in heavily trafficked areas and some are portable. You can also design a virtual bulletin board on the nursing professional development (NPD) website. Consider posting hypothetical case studies on bulletin boards. But don't put all of the information up at once. Start with learning objectives and an introduction to a case scenario, and end with a question that requires learners to do some investigating. That question can lead to the next segment of the bulletin board to be posted a week later. You could also offer a list of some journal articles or other resources to get them started.

- **Scavenger hunts:** This is a fun approach that can be part of mandatory training or any other educational event. In order to find clues, learners must read and evaluate a clinical situation. The clue involves determining a correct answer, such as reviewing lab results if an electrolyte imbalance is suspected. This would lead learners to visit the laboratory studies department to find the next clue. This approach, of course, involves getting permission and cooperation from departments who would house clues. The first person or team to solve the clinical scenario receives an award, such as a free meal in the cafeteria or other relatively inexpensive but fun prizes.

- **Journal clubs:** Journal clubs are generally used for teaching appraisal of research articles, describing innovations in diagnosis and treatment, and translating research findings into clinical practice application. Articles can be discussed at staff meetings but discussions are often more successful when conducted virtually. Post an article and a template for critiquing that article. Develop discussion questions. Make sure that the virtual journal club is password-protected and available only to employees. Send out e-mail or text announcements when new articles are posted. Set up opportunities for virtual discussion groups and ask for ideas for new articles.

- **Case studies:** These, too, can be designed for virtual implementation. Learners are usually most interested in topics that allow them to explore clinical practice and to identify best practice options.

The trick to searching for teaching options is to mix them up. For instance, suppose scavenger hunts are a big success for about a year, if that long. Then participation drops. This is because any strategy can become routine. Offer a limited number of events related to the same strategy and then discontinue them and try something new. Your learners will let you know when they want something reinstated.

19

Meeting the Demands of a One-Person NPD Department

It is important for all nursing professional development (NPD) specialists to stretch resources and find ways to eliminate unnecessary tasks; it is especially important for one-person NPD departments. Small departments are still called upon to meet the NPD needs of the nursing department as well as serve on a multitude of committees, act as change agents, and facilitate nursing practice. With limited NPD resources, one-person departments must be especially creative when it comes to surviving and thriving in the current healthcare environment. The following are some ideas to help manage your time and resources as a one-person department.

Eliminating Those "Extra" Tasks

It seems as though NPD departments have been assigned tasks that management or administration doesn't know what else to do with. Take a long, hard look at your responsibilities and identify those tasks that interfere with your ability to provide education and training. Gather evidence that documents how much time and what resources are used to fulfill these "extra" tasks. Document how this interferes with your ability to provide education, which you can note has a positive impact on job performance and patient outcomes.

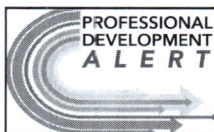

> **PROFESSIONAL DEVELOPMENT A L E R T** When proposing that you shed some of these "extra" tasks be sure to explain what you will do in place of them and how this will improve organizational effectiveness. You will also want to come up with recommendations as to how those tasks will be fulfilled (by someone else)!

Here are some examples of tasks that should not be your responsibility.

- Scheduling classroom, conference rooms, and A/V equipment. This is a serious waste of time. There are software programs that can facilitate scheduling and a reliable volunteer can help oversee this kind of issue. It is also a waste of money having a graduate-prepared NPD specialist do this work. Financial officers may get the idea that you can be replaced with someone much less expensive if this is one of the tasks that takes significant amounts of your time.

- Delivering A/V equipment and/or trouble-shooting problems with this equipment. You are not a delivery service. People reserving equipment should be responsible for picking it up. If the equipment is housed within the NPD department, you need to determine a centralized, safe location (e.g., the security office) to store a key to the equipment room. The key should be signed out and signed in as it is returned. You should not be expected to be "on-call" for equipment malfunction. People reserving the equipment are responsible for learning how to use it.

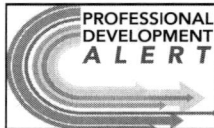

> **PROFESSIONAL DEVELOPMENT ALERT** As you abdicate responsibility for equipment it would be helpful to develop a list of trouble-shooting hints and attach these to the appropriate equipment. Such lists are usually available from the manufacturer.

- Coordinating Nurse Week activities or other social events. Such activities are not the responsibility of the NPD department. Nurse Week activities should be coordinated by a nursing committee. It seems that such social events are often assigned to the NPD department because "no one else has the time." If that is the excuse you are given, what does that say about how NPD services are viewed within your organization? If you hear this from others, you need to do a better job of presenting evidence regarding the impact of education.

- Serving on committees and task forces. Is there a link between these committees and education, or are you the go-to person for involvement because no one else has time? Again, if you are viewed as being the person with the most time to spare, that also means your position is the one most easily cut when budget deficits are looming.

These are just a few examples of tasks that interfere with delivery of NPD services. As a one-person department, you need to document evidence of your credibility as an education expert, not as someone who performs tasks that no one else wants to do.

Stretching Resources

How do you offer education on an ongoing basis when you are swamped by orientation, mandatory training, and accreditation preparation? The following are some suggestions for stretching the resources of a small department:

- Offer suggestions for healthcare mobile software applications (apps) that can be downloaded to smart phones or tablets. Make sure to preview and evaluate any app before recommending it. Also include if the app is free or if a charge is involved. Offering suggestions for apps as part of the education process helps cultivate self-direction and facilitates on-demand learning.

- Offer short bursts of learning sent directly to mobile devices. Collaborate with human resources to develop a database of contact numbers. Keeping this database current should be the responsibility of the learners. They must keep their information up to date and notify HR of any changes.

- Collaborate with local colleges and universities. Most faculty members need to publish and conduct research to advance professionally. By working with them, you can develop a variety of projects, especially those that are research-oriented.

- Contact your local chapter of Sigma Theta Tau International. Members are often interested in collaborating on education and research projects.

- Collaborate with managers of other disciplines. Interdisciplinary education and research offers benefits to all and enhances working relationships.

- Work with your information systems department to develop a professional development webpage as part of the hospital's intranet and Internet sites. Learners love the convenience of on-demand Internet learning. You can post education information on a variety of sources quickly and efficiently in this way.

- Be creative when using technology as a learning option. Don't just offer articles. Offer case studies that require some investigation on the part of the learner before solutions are revealed in a later posting. Use game formats such as crossword puzzles.

- Involve members of your education council and other councils if you are part of a shared governance system. If not, consider initiating an education committee.

- Check out the websites of your professional associations. Most of them have a discussion forum and opportunities to seek out mentors. Find out what your colleagues in similar positions are doing to alleviate the strain.

- If appropriate, collaborate with NPD colleagues locally and globally. You may be able to combine resources to offer in-person and distance learning activities that are valuable to all concerned. Be sure to check with your manager before initiating contact to avoid making any political faux pas.

- Make evidence-based practice the foundation of your NPD practice. You need to be able to show what you have accomplished and how collaboration or other innovative strategies can improve NPD services.

These ideas are not just for one-person departments. All of us are often stretched to the limits of time and resources. Be creative in your approach to education and collaborate whenever possible to maximize your time and talents!

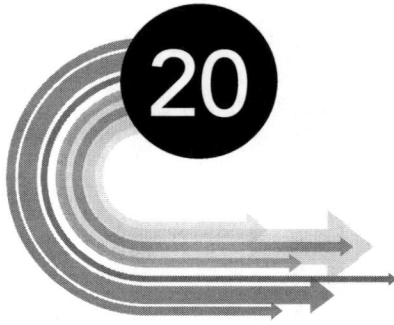

20 Assessing Literacy Levels

Preparing written materials for learners with various literacy levels can be problematic. We are responsible for providing education to people with varying levels of education and literacy. We also provide education for people for whom English is not a first language. Patient education materials must be at an appropriate reading level.

There is a lot to consider when developing written materials. Be sure to:

❑ Know your audience. Who will be using these materials? Tailor the handout to the learners' education and reading levels.

❑ Focus on critical concepts.

❑ Keep within a range of about a fourth to sixth grade reading level.

❑ Always pilot your materials before using them in education programs. Ask people in the target audience to review them for clarity and comprehension.

❑ Review sources of free materials that can be downloaded without copyright violation.

❑ Evaluate software programs that assess the reading levels of your written materials. Examples include: Center for Language Education and Research (CLEAR), Syllable Counter, SMOG Calculator, and Automated Readability Index (ARI).

❑ Review guidelines written by experts pertaining to literacy levels. Examples of such guidelines include:

  – MedlinePlus. (2009). How to write easy-to-read health materials. *www.nlm.nih.gov/medlineplus/etr.html.*

  – WordsCount. (2009). *www.wordscount.info/readability.html.*

  – UCDavis Health System. (2010). Guidelines for preparing patient education handouts. *www.ucdmc.ucdavis.edu/cne/health_education/guide.html.*

21

Writing Test Questions

Writing test questions is an acquired skill. Some programs, particularly programs that are certification related, come with tests already written. But we often need to develop our own test questions to assess learning. Most of us rely on multiple-choice questions. For the purpose of this chapter we will focus on multiple-choice items.

We need to develop questions that assess achievement of learning objectives, but are also easy to grade. We also need to avoid ambiguity and subjectivity. Carefully written multiple-choice questions seem to be the most efficient way of assessing learning in the written format.

Here are some guidelines for writing multiple-choice test questions:

- Multiple-choice questions consist of a question or an incomplete statement referred to as the "stem" of the question. The stem is followed by four choices, only one of which is the correct or best possible answer. Although NCLEX exam questions now offer answers such as "all of the above," or a combination of answers such as "a, b, and c," it is still recommended, in the professional setting, that only one choice is the best possible answer.

- Make sure that all of the four choices fit grammatically with the stem.

- Use simple sentence structure.

- Place most of the words in the stem of the question.

- Keep all answer choices the same length as much as possible. If this isn't possible, write two long and two short choices.

- Avoid double negatives and negative stem statements. Negatives are confusing.

- Mix up the order of the correct answers. For example, don't have the correct answers follow a logical path (e.g., the first question's correct answer is choice a, the second question's correct answer is b, and so on).

- Avoid using the same or similar words in both the stem and the correct answer (using the same words can give away the answer).

- Avoid options such as "none of the above," "some of the above," and "all of the above."

- Vary the complexity of the questions. For instance the simplest way to write a test question is to ask for a simple "knowledge" response. An example of this would be:

  Which of the following drugs depletes potassium?

  a. Lasix

  b. Amoxicillin

  c. Lipitor

  d. Benicar

A more advanced level of assessment would be to ask:

  Which of the following effects may occur in a patient taking large doses of Lasix on a daily basis?

  a. Hypokalemia

  b. Elevated WBC counts

  c. Hypercalcemia

  d. Decreased cholesterol

To respond appropriately the learner would have to know more about the impact of Lasix on a variety of lab results.

The way you write your stems should be based on your learning objectives and on the level of expertise of the learner. For example, the first example given is appropriate for a nursing student who is just beginning to learn about the principles of pharmacology. The second example is more appropriate for a professional nurse who should be able to differentiate among the affect of Lasix on a variety of lab studies.

Here are some good resources when writing test questions:

- Simple Guidelines for Writing Test Questions: *http://webs.rtc.edu/ii/Teaching%20Resources/ GuidelinesforWRitingTest.htm*

- Writing Instruction Objectives and Tests: *http://instructionaldesign.gordoncomputer.com/Objectives.html*

- 10 Rules for Writing Multiple Choice Questions: *http://thelearningcoach.com/elearning_design/ rules-for-multiple-choice-questions/*

22

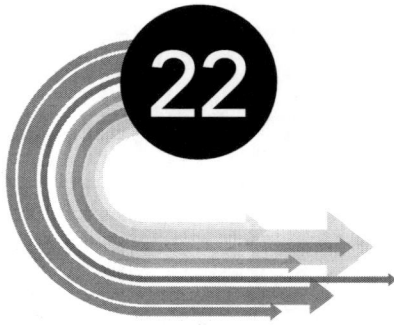

Facilitating Participation in Education

It has always been a challenge to release staff nurses from their duties at the bedside to participate in educational events. Distance education was supposedly going to be the answer to that problem, but what we have found that it is also a challenge for nurses to even find the time to access distance learning during the workday.

Nursing professional development (NPD) specialists assumed much of the burden (and the guilt) for lack of attendance. What we now know is that participation in education is part of a culture of learning, promoted by entities such as shared governance models and ANCC Magnet Recognition Program® (MRP) status.

Culture of Learning

What organizational model does your organization espouse? Are you part of a shared governance system with councils at unit-based and organizational levels? Does the phrase "culture of learning" appear in administrative documents, policies, and in verbal conversations? You are fortunate if you have a culture that supports learning and shared governance.

Any of these types of cultures is an emphasis on ongoing learning as part of a system that provides excellent patient care and has motivated, high-performing employees. Are beliefs in the importance of learning and education not only stated by administration, but operationalized? Administration should dedicate adequate financial and human resources for education and training.

Even if you are not part of a shared governance system, you need to promote a culture of learning, which is essential to education participation. Participation in such activities depends on:

- **Administrative and managerial support.** Job descriptions should contain mandates that all employees participate in a minimum number of educational events annually depending on roles and responsibilities. Managerial job descriptions should contain mandates stating that they and their nurses arrange scheduling to facilitate such attendance.

PROFESSIONAL
DEVELOPMENT
A L E R T

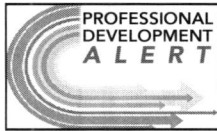

Adult learners are responsible for their own learning. As nurses become more and more em-powered at the staff nurse level, they must also assume responsibility for their own learning.

- **Dissemination of educational information.** NPD specialists must do more than simply publicize educa-tional events. We must provide evidence as to why participation is important and what impact education has on job performance and patient outcomes. As part of the announcement of educational events, we need to include whatever evidence we have as to the impact of such events. For example, if we are providing mock emergency drills, we should say how the drills have improved early recognition of deterioration of patients' conditions and how this recognition enhanced patient survival and patient outcomes. If we do not yet have that kind of data, we could provide information from the literature explaining how other organizations have improved outcomes after mock drills were initiated. We should also publicize not only learning objectives but overall goals, such as decreasing the number of deaths, transfers to critical care units, lengths of stay, etc. Our nursing colleagues, especially those from generation Y and beyond, are more likely to participate in education if they understand that education is linked to improved job performance, more positive patient outcomes, and the likelihood of career advancement.

- **Linking needs assessment data to learner outcomes and organizational goals.** Publicize how needs assessment data are used to plan and develop programs. Education council members should be intimately involved in bringing ideas, questions, and concerns from the units to the council; assisting with program planning and delivery; and participating in evaluating education outcomes. This is an excellent way to pro-mote the collaboration of staff nurses and NPD specialists in research projects linking the impact of educa-tion to clinical practice.

- **Offering education in a variety of formats.** We already know that a variety of formats and strategies is important. But we need to include format evaluation and attendance as part of our data analysis and docu-mentation of evidence. We need to determine what format seems to facilitate participation and if one format versus another has better impact on job performance and patient outcomes.

- **Recognition of successful education.** Recognize nurses and units that not only have the most evidence of education participation, but the most evidence that education participation led to positive results. For example, significant participation in programming related to communication and teamwork might lead to decreased turnover, increased retention, increased job satisfaction, fewer patient complaints, etc. Reward these nurses and/or units and recognize their contributions. Don't award so frequently that it becomes com-monplace and their impact is reduced. Rewards could be on an annual basis, perhaps during Nurse Week activities to keep it as a special type of recognition.

- **Promote the inclusion of "education participation time" as part of staff nurses' job responsibilities.** Nurses need to schedule education, whether it be classroom, simulation, computer-based learning, etc., just as they would schedule time to provide patient education, administer medications, or perform any other important duty. This scheduled time must be considered as important as any other responsibility; otherwise, nurses will always be "too busy."

A culture of learning means that education is recognized as important to the organization's effectiveness. It is imperative that we provide evidence that links education to this effectiveness. By showing the impact of education we can help to gain administrative buy-in for a true culture of learning.

23

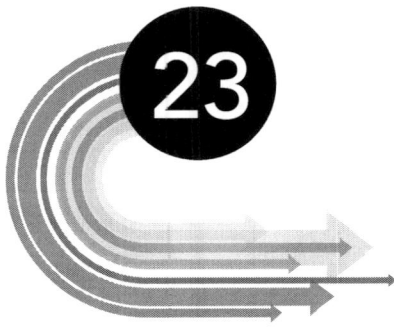

Using Apps as Teaching Interventions

The healthcare industry deals with constant, fast-paced change on what seems to be a daily basis. New ways of preventing, diagnosing, and treating diseases and injuries necessitate that those of us who work as healthcare professionals come to grips with the need to acquire new knowledge swiftly and efficiently. The only industry that equals, and may even surpass, the speed with which it experiences change is the technology industry. We have—at the touch of a button on a phone, computer, or tablet—access to amazing amounts of information.

As nursing professional development (NPD) specialists, we are always looking for ways to disseminate knowledge. Many of us have turned to mobile device software applications (or "apps") created for this new technology as a way to offer or facilitate education. However, our clinical nursing colleagues are already inundated with information. How do we evaluate the need to use apps and which apps to recommend?

Should I Use This App in My Teaching?

Remember, the primary reason to use an app as a teaching tool is because you consider it the best source of information and think it will enhance learning. Consideration of the following questions can help you determine whether to use an app:

- What is the purpose of using an app? Does it provide the best source of current information? Or are we simply trying to figuratively jump on the technology bandwagon and use a method we think will appeal to learners, especially learners who are enamored with this type of technology?

- How will we use the information acquired from an app? How does such information help achieve learning objectives?

- How will we know who has accessed the information from an app?

- How have we determined that all learners have access to the app we want to use? Not everyone has tools to access this type of technology (i.e., smartphones, tablets, etc.). Remember, some apps are only created for certain brands of mobile devices. We also cannot mandate a tool that requires learners to incur unnecessary expense.

Incorporating an App Into Teaching Strategy

If you have determined that an app will be part of your teaching strategy, you need to decide how you are going to incorporate it. The following are some factors to consider:

- You should identify the purpose of the app in relation to learning objectives.

- If there is a cost related to using the app? If so, who is going to assume the burden of payment? Have you incorporated this cost into your budget? Is the app a mandatory part of the learning experience or simply recommended? If only recommended, you need to ensure that all learners, even those who do not access the app, receive similar information. If they don't have access to the app, how will learners achieve learning objectives?

- How are you going to assess if learners have access to the app? Will this be a prerequisite to the class? How can you make information available to learners who do not have access to the app? You need to evaluate if access to an app is essential or just nice to have.

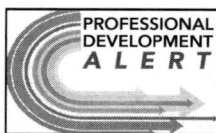

PROFESSIONAL DEVELOPMENT ALERT Don't mandate information from an app just to attract learners. There must be a valid reason to use it.

Including an App as Part of a Resource List

Rather than mandating an app, you may want to consider identifying appropriate apps as part of a resource list, the same way you would include books, DVDs, etc., in a resource list. When compiling a list of apps to use as resource information, include the following information as part of the listings:

- ❑ **Cost.** Explain whether the app is free. If there is a cost, identify the cost and whether there are additional costs to update the app.

- ❑ **Disclaimer.** Learners will expect that you evaluate the quality of the app; however, you need to include a statement such as, "The information regarding cost and quality of information is current as of [insert date]. Remember that cost and quality may change without warning."

- ❑ **Instructions.** Include how to download the app, and include all brand-specific information.

Evaluate every app you place on a resource list! Never recommend an app without evaluating it. When evaluating an app be sure to assess:

- ❏ Cost of initial download

- ❏ Cost of updates

- ❏ Source of app

- ❏ Whether the information provided by the app is current and kept updated

- ❏ Whether the information provided by the app is accurate

- ❏ Whether the app can be used on all types of mobile devices, or just certain brands

Suggested Apps

Here are a few apps that you may find useful. Just type the names of the app as listed into your app search engine or market. However, remember to evaluate them for yourself. As already noted, cost and quality can change without notice.

- **AHRQePSS:** The Electronic Preventive Services Selector (EPSS) is designed by the U.S. Department of Health & Human Services' Agency for Healthcare Research and Quality. The app was developed to help primary care clinicians identify screening, counseling, and preventive medication services for patients.

- **AUDIO- Medical Spanish (EMSG):** This emergency medical Spanish guide is designed for non-Spanish speaking healthcare professionals to obtain necessary medical information.

- **Black's Medical Dictionary:** This app allows access to the best-selling medical dictionary for more than 100 years. Provides clear explanations of medical terms.

- **Blausen Human Atlas:** Animated illustrations and three-dimensional rotating body systems in one app.

- **CCRN Exam Prep:** Upward Mobility's CCRN app is designed to help prepare nurses for the American Association of Critical Care Nurses' critical care certification exam.

- **Continuing Education Trackers:** Tracks license and certification renewals, professional courses, expenses, and required continuing education hours.

- **Dosage Calc:** Assists in drug calculations.

© 2012 HCPro, Inc.

- **IV Drug Handbook:** Offers practical guidelines pertaining to administration of intravenous drugs.

- **MedCalc 3000 Complete:** This is the most popular medical calculator system on the Web as of this writing.

- **Medscape:** Medscape provides information on every conceivable drug and disease. Also includes up-to-the-minute news about breaking research findings.

- **Nurse's Pocket Drug Guide 6th Edition:** Provides information on 1,000 commonly used medications.

- **Pocket EKG-Basic:** Helps you to interpret the 25 most common cardiac dysrhythmias. An interactive quiz is included.

24

Ineffective Guest Educators

Sooner or later we all face the uncomfortable prospect of dealing with an ineffective guest educator. As a guest, he or she is not a member of the nursing professional development (NPD) department (and may not even be an employee of your organization). The guest is offering time and expertise to meet some type of learning need. However, evaluations rate the guest as poor and learners complain about the educator's teaching style.

Before we fire the guest, it is important to evaluate the actual effectiveness (or lack of effectiveness) of our guest. We also need to consider the political ramifications of discontinuing a working relationship with this educator. It is extremely difficult and uncomfortable to tell the director of nursing or a prominent physician that his or her services are no longer needed by the department. It may also be political suicide. How can we determine if this relationship is salvageable? How can we help guest educators to improve their teaching skills?

We need to start by gathering and analyzing evidence pertaining to the guest's teaching effectiveness. Gathering and analyzing evidence is the cornerstone of NPD evidence-based practice (EBP).

Reaction Data

What do the reaction-related data from the evaluations tell us about the guest educator's teaching effectiveness? Analyze comments objectively. Are learners basically complaining about presentation style? For example, do the learners perceive the guest educator as boring? Do they complain about not being able to hear him or her? Are they having trouble hearing or seeing audiovisual aids?

These kinds of comments describe issues that can tactfully be addressed with (most) guest educators. Eliminate comments that are downright rude and focus first on the educator's strengths and then discuss the issues that need to be resolved to enhance presentation effectiveness. You may want to share some areas that you personally had to improve in and how you did so. Stress that you are still interested in having the guest participate, but want the experience to be valuable for all concerned.

Before inviting guest educators to present content, let them know that learners will be evaluating them. Make sure that they are involved in determining the learning objectives and identifying how achievement of those objectives will be evaluated. Give them a copy of the blank evaluation template so they understand what is meant by evaluation. Share the different levels of evaluation with them and explain how data from the different levels are used. Prepare them to anticipate being evaluated.

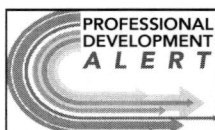

> **PROFESSIONAL DEVELOPMENT ALERT** If you anticipate that discussing areas for improvement may trigger political ramifications, you'll want to alert your manager before any discussions take place.

Learning Data

Learning is part (or should be part) of every education experience. Ensure that there is a learning component to your guest educators' presentations. It could be a post-test, quiz, skill demonstration, critical thinking exercise, etc. When you analyze the data from the learning component of learner evaluations, questions you should answer include:

- Did participants learn what they were supposed to learn?

- Did they achieve the learning objectives?

If the answer to these questions is "yes," you need to ask yourself if the poor evaluations are reactive in nature and reflect dissatisfaction with presentation style. If learning is achieved, then work to help the guest educators enhance their ability to present. It may be that you are willing to put up with speakers who are, quite frankly, rather boring, as long as participants are learning. Some people are nationally recognized experts and possess amazing amounts of knowledge, but are not the best presenters; however, they may still be the best available resources you have.

But, if learning is not taking place, your problem is more serious than simply improving presentation style. Answer these questions.

- Why isn't learning taking place? Did content not correlate with learning objectives?

- Did the guest fail to comprehend what the content was to be in relationship to learning objectives?

- Did the educator deliberately choose not to include agreed upon content? If so, why did this occur?

- Did you and the guest educator spend adequate time discussing learning objectives and what needed to be included to achieve those objectives prior to presentation?

You need to share learning data with your guest educators. These types of data may have more of an impact than reaction data. The more objective evidence you are able to compile, the more objective your suggestion is for revisions to the guest educator's content and/or presentation style.

Behavior Data

Analysis of behavioral data in your evaluations seeks to establish an association between education and changes in the behavior in learners. In other words, you are looking for evidence that the education has made a positive difference in behavior. Examples include changes in, or applications of, a new documentation system, procedure, or communication technique. Providing behavioral evidence usually has even more of an impact on your guest educator than reaction and learning data.

Results and Return on Investment Data

If you can tie in education provided by guest educators to results and return on investment (ROI), by all means do so. The more objective evidence you can provide the better. To be able to explain to guest educators that they helped to decrease infection rates or lengths of stay, or saved a specific amount of money thanks to a decrease in turnover, is a powerful motivator to do their best as educators.

Tips for Talking to Guest Educators

When talking to guest educators, remember that the guest may also be concerned about his or her performance as an educator. Try the following tips:

- Start by sharing the positive data from evaluations and any evidence that links their efforts to learning, behavior, results, and/or ROI.

- Always come prepared with suggestions on how they can improve their role as educators. Don't simply present negative findings without some ideas on how these can be improved.

- Alert your manager if you anticipate that there may be political ramifications to discussions related to the effectiveness of particular guest educators. Do this before you talk to the guest educators.

- Consider team-teaching as an alternative to having a guest speaker present alone. This may help to reduce some negative reaction data by reducing the time the guest actually presents.

- Consider incorporating some distance learning concepts for guest educators who have knowledge to share but do not particularly like to present before a live audience. They may enjoy preparing written case studies or a slide deck rather than actually committing time and effort to presenting live.

Some guest educators may be offended and unable to take constructive criticism. They may choose to stop participating in your education efforts. If this is the case, you may be better off without their assistance. Don't take such reactions personally. The guest educators may actually be looking for a way to avoid presenting and negative evaluations may provide them with a reason to leave under their own conditions.

Finally, some learners may question why that boring guest is still part of the education for your organization. Don't be afraid to share positive evidence that learners are acquiring and applying knowledge learned from that particular speaker. Also, you can share with learners that you and the guest speaker are working to improve those areas that have caused dissatisfaction.

25

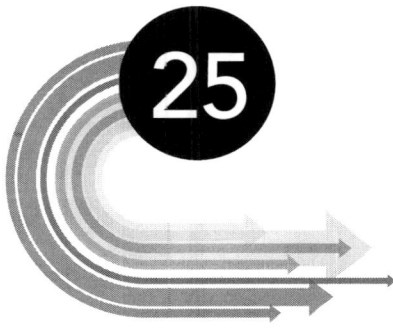

Teaching New Graduates Versus Experienced Nurses

Our learners represent a wide variety of experience levels. We often develop a program that both newly licensed nurses and nurses with many years of experience attend. How can we keep from overwhelming some and boring others?

When planning education programs think about where and how you can add additional resources for people needing some background information. For the typical continuing education program, it is nearly impossible to plan and implement more than one version of the program, even though you might like to be able to spend more time on basic concepts with some learners and add more sophisticated information for others.

Sample Scenario

Let's follow a hypothetical example of a series of continuing education activities designed for physical rehabilitation nurses. The scenario involves a group of nurses of various levels of experience. The organization in which they work is trying to achieve designation as a stroke center. In order to accomplish this goal, nurses need to be educated regarding emergency and acute care of the stroke patient, rehabilitation of the stroke patient, and discharge planning including prevention and follow-up care.

Start by identifying classes that are important for all nurses. Pathophysiology of stroke and physical assessment are important topics for nurses at all points in the care continuum and may be appropriate for a blended learning or all-distance learning approach. The pathophysiology component could include resource materials such as additional journal articles, a vocabulary list, and website referrals. Some nurses will need to access these resources, others will not. The point is that nurses who are not as familiar with stroke pathophysiology will have additional resources to help define and explain some sophisticated content.

For those nurses who are more familiar with the topic, these resources are not necessary. For these more experienced nurses, compile a list of more sophisticated resources. You may want to identify the resources as basic and advanced information so that nurses can access what they need. Some computer-based learning (CBL) programs offer the learner the opportunity to click on words that they need defined or to access practice items. These options are excellent ways to offer additional tutoring without mandating that all nurses avail themselves of the opportunity. As long as learning objectives and achievement measurements are made clear, it is up to the learner to determine the type of resources her or she needs to access.

The next step is to identify classes that will be offered according to specialty. Emergency measures are not mandated for rehabilitation nurses, and rehabilitation initiatives are not mandatory for emergency nurses. Focus can be broken into specialties. Within those specialties the same concept of offering resources that vary in sophistication is applicable.

When incorporating psychomotor skill components of classes, make sure that you allow for practice time. For example, nurses who have had stroke rehabilitation experience are more likely to be ready to demonstrate transfer techniques sooner than nurses who are new to the specialty of stroke rehabilitation. Don't make the nurses who are ready to demonstrate competency practice a specified number of times. Let them pursue return demonstration as soon as possible. For nurses who need time to absorb the skill, allow practice time away from those nurses who are ready to demonstrate competency. Don't make it a race. Nothing makes some people more uncomfortable than feeling we are the last to grasp something new.

Do not, however, divide the class into groups of "experienced" versus "new" nurses. They can learn from each other. Experienced nurses can share their knowledge and newer nurses bring fresh perspectives.

Advance Preparation

Prior to any education that is required or part of an important organizational goal, provide information about where nurses can access information prior to attending education. Although some nurses certainly will not prepare in advance, you may be surprised at the number of nurses who will appreciate having you guide them to materials that will help them prepare for class. This is especially true if resources are made available electronically. A click of the mouse allows them to access journal articles from the organization's library. Or, if your organization does not have that capability, provide a list of resources and direction on how to obtain them.

Ongoing Learning

Ideally, adult learners recognize their own learning needs and seek out opportunities to grow professionally. In reality, however, nurses are more likely to seek out opportunities that are easy to access. As nursing professional development (NPD) specialists, we need to help nurses identify learning resources. Some NPD specialists have identified resources and made lists available on units, on the NPD website, etc., and specified skill levels of these resources.

For instance, nurses just beginning to learn about the nursing research process would appreciate information on how to conduct literature searches, critique research articles, etc. Nurses who already have some research experience need more sophisticated materials, such as articles on how to select appropriate research methods and/or identify appropriate methods of statistical analysis. By identifying the level of sophistication of resources, you are helping learners avoid becoming overwhelmed or bored.

Simulation

One of the best ways to meet the needs of learners with a variety of expertise is simulation. Remember that simulation can take many forms, not just using sophisticated equipment. Role-play, mock drills, and interactive theater all allow for nurses from all backgrounds to work together to create "real-life" experiences in a nonthreatening environment. For more information regarding simulation, refer to Chapter 13 on simulation.

Case Studies

Case studies are a terrific strategy for meeting the needs of learners with various skill levels. You can write and upload (or distribute hard copies of) case studies that rely on clinical scenarios as a teaching tool. These scenarios can be written to meet the needs of learners new to a specialty or the practice of nursing, or nurses who are experts in their fields. Again, clearly identify the complexity of each case study so that learners can choose where to start and advance at their own pace.

These are just a few ideas. Ask learners for their suggestions as well.

26

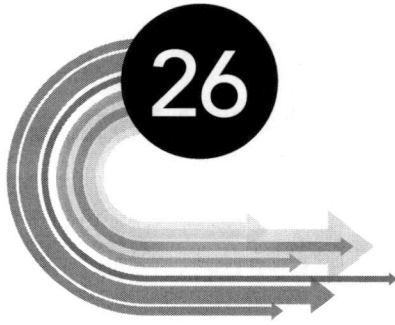

Teaching Learners From Different Generations

There are many different generations in the workplace today. Nurses and other healthcare professionals are living longer and retiring later. Some of our older colleagues continue to serve in healthcare as volunteers. Our youngest colleagues represent a generation born with the world virtually at their fingertips.

Teaching members of four to five generations at one time in the same learning environment causes a number of challenges. The following are some ideas for teaching members of different generations (Avillion, 2008).

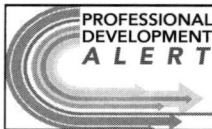

> **PROFESSIONAL DEVELOPMENT ALERT**
>
> These suggestions are broad guidelines. All learners are unique and may vary in characteristics. Also, the years of birth for each generation may vary depending on what resource you consult.

Veterans/Traditionalists

Born between 1926 and 1945, veterans or traditionalists generally grew up in what was once the traditional nuclear family consisting of two parents and their children. The father generally provided the income and the mother did not work outside the home. These learners generally prefer a more formal learning environment and often view educators as authority figures. When teaching veterans/traditionalists:

- Make sure that learning objectives and how they are to be achieved are clearly stated and understood.

- When using distance learning, make it clear where and how learners should go for help with new or unfamiliar technology.

- Provide organized, clearly stated handouts that summarize key points of the educational activity.

- Avoid small print when developing handouts or selecting fonts for computer-based learning. Don't use any font size less than 12 points and use fonts that are easy to read, such as Arial.

- Avoid asking them to demonstrate new or unfamiliar techniques in front of a group unless they have had an opportunity to practice first.

- Treat them with respect at all times. Acknowledge their life experiences.

- Never presume that members of this generation are technology-illiterate.

- Motivate these learners by explaining how education will improve job performance or volunteer experiences.

- Members of this generation are unlikely to confront you in person, so encourage feedback during breaks or midway through a learning activity.

Baby Boomers

Baby boomers, born between 1946 and 1964, grew up believing that they were entitled to the best the world had to offer. They highly value teamwork and personal gratification in the workplace. Boomers have a strong work ethic. When teaching members of this generation:

- Correlate education activities with improved job performance and opportunities for promotion.

- Incorporate interactive educational activities, such as icebreakers.

- Incorporate team-building activities as part of education.

- Avoid role-playing as the sole means of education. Boomers do not especially like role-play but are becoming more comfortable with the concept as simulation grows in acceptance and sophistication.

- Make sure that information is easily accessible. Remember that this was the first generation to make extensive use of the Internet.

- Avoid small print. Use at least a 12-point font and easy-to-read font such as Arial.

Generation X

Generation X was born between 1965 and 1980. They were the first generation to view the trend of single-parent families as the norm and use of the computer as part of everyday life. Xers are also known as the latch-key generation, with both parents working outside the home or the single-parent working outside the home. They have seen their parents experience downsizing and this was the first generation whose loyalty was to their career and themselves and not to an organization. Xers are cautious about money and view education as a means to achieve success.

Having seen their parents, the baby boomers, spend long hours at work during the week and on weekends, they seek a balance between work and leisure activity. When teaching Xers remember:

- Incorporate fun as part of learning. Xers value fun as part of learning activities.

- Offer hands-on learning activities. Xers learn best by doing and enjoy role-playing.

- Allow plenty of time for discussion, or for distance learning activities, adequate means of asking questions and expressing concerns (e.g., texting, e-mail).

- Demonstrate your expertise and share your enthusiasm. You need to earn the respect of Xers; it is not automatically bestowed just because someone holds a supervisory position.

- Include lots of visual stimulation such as tables, graphs, and illustrations. Xers, unlike boomers, do not especially enjoy reading.

Generation Y

Generation Y was born between 1981 and 2002. They grew up with technology and can't imagine a world without computers, social networking, and smart phones. They are globally oriented and move, think, and talk at top speed. Having witnessed the downsizing phenomenon become the norm for their parents, Yers have even less company loyalty than Xers. When teaching Yers:

- Provide opportunities for personal interaction with learning. Yers are so accustomed to technology that the opportunity to talk face-to-face is special.

- Include both structure and fun as part of learning activities.

- Expect education to be on-demand and offered at times convenient to them.

- Offer opportunities to participate in mentor programs.

- Explain how education can increase job performance and opportunities for promotion.

- Offer lists of reading resources. Yers enjoy reading.

The Path to Stress-Free Nursing Professional Development

Generation Z

The next generation to enter the workplace, born anywhere between the late 1990s and early 2000s (depending on what resource you use), have yet to enter the workplace. However, we can make some educated guesses about their characteristics.

Generation Z not only relies on the latest technology, but expect to update the technology they do have on an almost ongoing basis. Interacting globally is the norm and they want everything from education to communication to shopping to happen instantly. So much of their communication is online or via texting that there is legitimate concern about their ability to acquire interpersonal, face-to-face communication skills, which is so important to patient interaction.

It is anticipated that education will need to be not only flexible and on-demand but updated quickly. They will not tolerate outdated information (and outdated may mean months or even weeks instead of years). They expect that simulation be frequently part of learning and they value fun and physical activity as part of learning. We will also need to stress communication and should be prepared to address issues such as body language and verbal and nonverbal communication as part of most learning activities.

In summary, NPD specialists must be prepared to move at lightning speed while monitoring learning among participants who come from distinct generational perspectives. Stress the opportunities for learning from each other and creativity at all times.

Reference

Avillion, A. E. (2008). *A Practical Guide to Staff Development: Evidence-based Tools and Techniques for Effective Education.* Danvers, MA: HCPro, Inc.

27

Teaching the Art of Conducting a Literature Review

As staff nurses assume more and more responsibility for evidence-based practice and participating in research, it is imperative that they be able to conduct a literature review and critique journal articles. Nurses are often asked to perform a literature review without any guidelines. Some of them may assume that because an article has been published, it is credible. But this is certainly not the case, particularly for articles published on independent websites.

You need to give staff nurses who are embarking on their first research initiatives or participating on councils as part of shared governance guidelines for literature review. Here are some suggested guidelines to help you get started:

- Most nurses will start their literature review with an Internet search. This is okay as long as they know how to do it. Help them to clarify what they are going to type in their search browsers. For instance, if they are investigating urinary tract infections associated with catheterization, they shouldn't simply type in "urinary tract infections." They need to refine their search. They might narrow it by typing in "urinary tract infections due to catheterization" or, to narrow it even further, "nosocomial urinary tract infections due to catheterization." Help them to clarify what their goal is.

- When evaluating articles, teach them to first evaluate the source. Is the article from a credible professional journal? If the article is taken from a website, is the source credible? For example, is the website a personal website or from a recognized, credible source such as the Mayo Clinic? If the article is not from a credible, professional source, it should be eliminated from the literature review at this time.

- Who are the authors of the articles? What are their credentials? Is professional contact information for the authors listed? Most credible journals and websites list author credentials as well as their professional affiliations. Do credentials and professional affiliations indicate expertise in the content of the article?

- What is the publication date of the article? Remember that it may take one or more years from the time an article is submitted for publication to the time it is actually published. Based on the time frame from submission to publication, the information contained in the article may be out of date.

- Are references listed for each article? Are these references credible and timely?

- Is the research question clearly stated? If not, the article should be discounted. If yes, does the article address the question the authors set out to answer?

- Is the theoretical framework for the research design described? Is the research based on valid and reliable frameworks that are relevant to the research question?

- Is the research method appropriate? This may be difficult for nurses to answer based on their level of expertise. Help them to look for associations between how the research was conducted and the actual research question.

- How were data collected? Were tools used that are valid and reliable? If the authors developed the research tool, how did they test it for validity and reliability?

- What was the sample size? Just because the size is small does not mean the article is inadequate. But, if it is small, how do the authors address the issue of a small sample size?

- How were participants selected for inclusion in the study? Were they (ideally) selected at random? Is there any indication of bias in participate selection?

- What are the limitations of the study? Are they identified by the authors? How do the authors address identified limitations?

- What conclusions are made by the authors? Do these conclusions make sense? Are they based on objective analysis of data? Are the conclusions supported by the data?

- Have the authors identified implications for further research? This is important because it means the authors have considered the implications of their study and recognize the need for more study.

- Have the authors clearly identified implications for patient outcomes and/or professional practice?

- Do the authors have a commercial interest in research outcomes or indicate any bias? If the answer to either question is "yes," that could indicate that the research might not be objective.

These guidelines should be reviewed with staff nurses prior to expecting them to conduct literature reviews. They need to be able to gather relevant resources, especially as clinical research—starting with the staff nurse at the patient bedside—is gaining prominence and importance.

28

Evaluating Healthcare Websites

The Internet is a source of infinite information for healthcare professionals and healthcare consumers. However, because of the sheer volume of information, it is impossible to monitor the accuracy of content. As nursing professional development (NPD) specialists, we are often called upon to help nursing staff evaluate the reliability of healthcare websites. We are also frequently asked to help develop guidelines for patients and families who may believe anything and everything they read online. How can we help others to differentiate the reliable from the inaccurate, and from the just plain wrong?

Staff members and patients/families may benefit from receiving a list of healthcare websites that you have evaluated and determined to be accurate and reliable; however, we can't continually review information every day for accuracy and reliability and do not want to be legally and ethically responsible for approving website content. If you choose to provide such a list, make sure that you include a disclaimer stating that the websites listed have been found to provide healthcare information that is generally reliable, but reliability and accuracy cannot be guaranteed because content may change without warning. You should also add that patients should never alter their prescribed treatment based on website content. Questions and concerns should always be directed to their healthcare providers.

Encourage patients to print information from websites and bring it with them to appointments with their healthcare providers for review and clarification. Even referring patients to your organization's website may have legal ramifications because you don't have control over every aspect of content. The organization's education council or similar committee may want to make review of the organization's website teaching materials an objective.

Origin of Website

What is the source of the website? Is it run by an organization or by an individual? If it is sponsored by an organization the reliability of the organization must be assessed.

What type of organization is responsible for the website? Is it a professional healthcare organization? If so, does the organization have a good professional reputation that is regionally or nationally recognized? For example, the Mayo Clinic has a worldwide reputation for healthcare excellence. If information is being retrieved from a local healthcare facility, does that facility have a reputation for excellence? Does your own organization have a website with information for healthcare professionals and/or consumers? Do you feel comfortable recommending information from your organization's website?

> **PROFESSIONAL DEVELOPMENT ALERT**
>
> If you don't feel comfortable recommending your own organization's website you need to do something about it. If you are aware of inaccuracies you have a professional obligation to initiate corrections. Your organization's website is a good way to provide various types of education for staff members and patients/families. As an educator, you should be involved in the way education materials are presented.

Is the website owned, operated, and or maintained by a for-profit company such as a publishing house or pharmaceutical company? If so, does the website identify any bias or commercial interest that may have that have an influence over what is published and how it is published? Caution people who access such sites to be aware of these issues. For example, a pharmaceutical firm may be heavily biased in favor of a drug it developed for treatment of a certain disease and use its website to extol the virtues of that drug without mentioning other treatment options. This is a good way to teach learners not to rely on one source of information, but instead to consult a variety of reputable sources when researching a patient care issue or, in the case of patients/families, treatment options.

Is the site owned and/or operated by an individual versus an organization? Remember that anyone can set up a website and pretty much say whatever they want. It is easy to access information published online by a patient who wants to relay his or her own experiences. Some of this type of information is heavily biased and the website may be used to vent frustration and anger. Some individuals may want to share more positive experiences and discuss treatment options that worked for them. If this type of information triggers questions and concerns, that is okay as long as the reader who is a healthcare professional seeks out scientifically valid information as well and the reader who is a patient takes concerns to his or her healthcare provider.

Be wary of relying on information supplied by a consumer who has no credentials to support conclusions or recommendations! Many people, both healthcare professionals and consumers alike, become caught up in the emotion of a story rather than objectively evaluate its validity.

Does the site contain commercial advertising? What products does the site endorse? Do these products indicate a bias for or against any treatment options or healthcare-related options? If bias exists, information should be reviewed with caution.

Does the website have an identified purpose? Is the purpose technical, scholarly, commercial, or social? Or is there a combination of purposes? Healthcare professionals conducting literature reviews or scholarly research should avoid social networking websites.

Authorship

Who is responsible for the maintenance of the website? Are the authors involved in its maintenance? How often is the site updated and by whom? Some sites contain excellent articles and/or links but, when carefully reviewed, are found to be quite outdated. Always check the date that information was secured for publication, written, or reviewed.

What are the authors' credentials, background, and expertise? Are they qualified to write, research, or otherwise comment on the information they have posted, published, or discussed? Have they posted written disclaimers stating that they are free from commercial bias? If such bias exists, how have they ensured the objectivity of their work? Is their work timely and relevant? What resources and references have the authors used in their work? Are these resources and references timely and free of commercial bias?

Content

Are publications and/or postings well written? If research is being presented, is the research design sound? Are there any obvious omissions or errors in the content, such as citing drugs that have been removed from the market by the U.S. Food and Drug Administration (FDA) as treatment options? Is the content based on scientific fact and evidence-based practice, or is it filled with opinions unsupported by data?

HON

Health on the Net Foundation (HON) is a nongovernment organization founded to "encourage the dissemination of quality health information for patients and professionals and the general public and to facilitate access to the latest and most relevant medical data through the use of the Internet" (*www.healthonnet.org*).

The HON code is used by more than 7,300 certified websites, more than 10 million pages, and in more than 100 countries. To qualify for certification, websites must:

1. List qualifications of authors.

2. Note that information provided is given to support, not replace, information given by patients' healthcare providers.

3. Ensure that the privacy of site users is respected.

4. Cite sources and dates of medical information.

5. Justify claims with objective data.

6. Provide valid contact details with accessible information.

7. Disclose details of financial funding.

8. Clearly distinguish advertising from editorial content.

It may be worthwhile to check if websites you are viewing are certified by HON. Visit the HON website for further information.

The preceding issues are just some of the considerations that healthcare professionals and consumers must think about when accessing healthcare websites. Before using any information published on the Internet, be sure to evaluate it carefully using the questions posed in this chapter as guidelines.

Communication

Learning Objective

- Implement education strategies to enhance communication in healthcare organizations.

Section 2

29

Conflict Resolution

Conflict in the workplace is an ongoing problem. As nursing professional development (NPD) specialists, we encounter conflict from many sources: employees who are resistant to learning, managers who resent when education requires staff nurses to be away from patient care, and colleagues who are resistant to changes that require education and training. The first step in conflict resolution is to recognize what factors contribute to conflict. Some of these factors are (Scott, 2010):

- **Differences in values.** Values are intertwined with moral and ethical beliefs. When an issue occurs that threatens a person's values, conflict occurs. For example, learners may believe that a change in policy or procedure will interfere with their ability to provide safe and appropriate nursing care. Their values as nurses may be threatened in this case.

- **Fear.** Fear manifests itself in many ways. Fear of change. Fear that someone or something may place a job in jeopardy. Fear of competition. Fear is a powerful motivator when it comes to conflict.

- **Miscommunication.** No matter how clearly we think we communicate, miscommunication is always a possibility, whether verbally or in writing. For example, we may state that a learning objective is to successfully demonstrate safe and accurate administration of medications during a mock cardiac arrest scenario. Further explanation may include the statement that critical care nurses must pass this skill demonstration before administering medications during an actual code. Some employees interpret this as meaning they may not work at all until they pass the skill demonstration. Such misunderstanding or lack of clarity can set up a massive conflict.

- **Treatment of others.** How we treat one another can alleviate or trigger conflict. Memories of prior conflicts may trigger new ones. Previous concerns or issues of mistrust may also trigger conflict.

- **Honesty.** Even though you may have always been honest in dealing with colleagues, they may have memories of others in positions of authority who have been dishonest or who have not always been frank in their dealings with others. This type of breach of trust triggers powerful feelings of betrayal and conflict often results.

- **Attitudes.** Attitudes are difficult to objectively measure. Although negative attitudes are often blamed for conflict, this is not necessarily true. We must consider all possible sources of conflict. However, there are those employees whose attitude predisposes conflict. These are employees who are not motivated to resolve conflict, who seek only to win at the expense of others or the organization.

Recognizing the particular source or sources that influence your interactions with others helps us to understand what is triggering the conflict. Now you need to determine what strategy to use to resolve the conflict. The four basic strategies are (McVay, 2007):

- **Accommodation:** Giving the other person or group what they want.

- **Assertion:** Concern for self is the priority with little or no concern for others, the organization, or, in the case of healthcare professionals, the patient. Also referred to as win/lose.

- **Avoidance:** Conflict is completely avoided or ignored. The hope is that the problem will resolve itself or just disappear.

- **Negotiation:** Conflict is resolved to the satisfaction of everyone involved. Also referred to as win/win.

Usually negotiation is the most desirable strategy. Avoidance is rarely effective unless the problem is deemed unworthy of investing time and energy for resolution. An example might be a disagreement over who gets to go to lunch early. If it's a one-time issue, it may be best to just let it go.

Assertion is usually a poor option, particularly when it compromises patient care. However, assertion is appropriate when an immediate decision is required without negotiation. Examples of this include emergency situations when swift decisions must be made and are not open to discussion (unless someone is performing an action that endangers patients).

Accommodation is also a strategy that is seldom effective unless the issue is quite trivial. The old saying about picking your battles is often true. Save your energy to resolve those conflicts that affect patient care and organizational or departmental effectiveness.

Steps for conflict resolution include:

1. Identify the most probable cause of conflict. Go beyond the overt issue (e.g., staff who don't want a new system of scheduling, or think they have no time to attend mandatory training, etc.) and look at underlying reasons such as fear, miscommunication, and dishonesty.

2. Decide which of the four strategies to choose. Ask yourself if the issue at hand is truly a conflict or just a minor annoyance. Whenever possible, work at negotiation so that everyone involved feels at least some degree of satisfaction in knowing that the best decision was reached for the well-being of the patients and the organization.

There may be instances in which there is little time to prepare a resolution. For example, you may be confronted by an angry employee who has failed to achieve a critical competency. You need to make a quick assessment about underlying causes and appropriate strategies. If the issue is one that allows you time to set up a meeting (e.g., meeting with nurse managers to solve preceptor dilemmas) you will have more time to prepare. If you have the luxury of time, use it.

If you have the time:

❏ Acknowledge the differences of opinion and that everyone's viewpoints are respected.

❏ Describe the conflict and its impact on job performance and patient care.

❏ Identify the goals that the involved parties hope to achieve. Always stress that the ultimate goal is to improve patient care and organizational effectiveness.

❏ Ask for and listen to proposed resolutions from all involved parties.

❏ Listen actively. Maintain eye contact and present an open body language. (For more on body language see Chapter 30 on enhancing communication skills.)

❏ Ask for clarification if you don't understand the point someone is trying to make.

❏ Ask if others need clarification of your point of view.

❏ Select a private, comfortable space to discuss resolution of conflict. Don't allow a scene in a public area.

❑ Avoid using language that places blame such as, "You don't return my phone calls," "You don't understand how important it is that your nurses attend this education program," or "You are not supporting my orientation program." Instead:

– Focus on the issue, not the person. For instance, discuss the best approach to facilitate and improve the preceptor program instead of asking why the preceptors on a unit are not properly orienting new nurses.

– Use "I" language. For example, "I would like to discuss how we can facilitate attendance at mandatory education programs," or "I feel it would be helpful to review the current orientation program and discuss how we can best orient our new nurses."

– Conclude by summarizing what you've agreed upon and how this agreement will improve job performance, patient care, and/or organizational effectiveness.

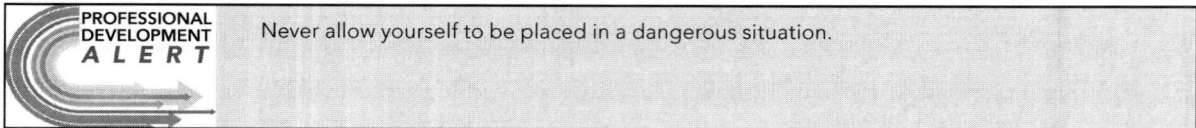

> **PROFESSIONAL DEVELOPMENT ALERT** Never allow yourself to be placed in a dangerous situation.

Be wary of dangerous situations. For example, if you are dealing with an angry colleague, make sure that you have a clear exit from the room in which you are meeting. Don't allow the angry person to get between you and the exit. If you know in advance that a meeting might become especially contentious, tell a colleague where and when you are meeting and make sure you meet in a location that has an easy exit and readily available assistance. Don't be afraid to call for help if you need it!

References

McVay, S. (2007). Conflict resolution: Turning a negative into a positive. *LPN*, 3(2), 9-10.

Scott, V. (2010). *Conflict Resolution at Work for Dummies.* Hoboken, NJ: Wiley Publishing.

30

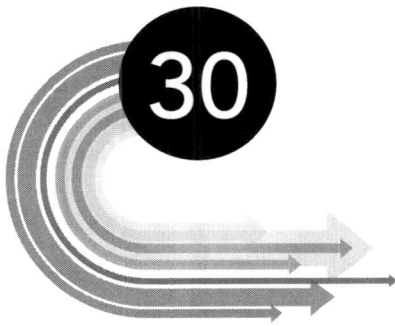

Enhancing Communication Skills

Most, if not all, nursing professional development (NPD) specialists can explain the principles and behaviors of good communication. Most healthcare professionals probably can, too. Why, then, is communication such an issue? How can we teach communication skills more effectively?

We'll begin by reviewing good communication skills and then move on to describe some innovative strategies for teaching such skills.

Review of Good Communication Skills

Good communication skills include the following:

❑ Maintain a calm tone of voice. Don't shout and don't whisper. Speak in a tone that is audible and clear.

❑ Avoid slang and acronyms. Not everyone understands the same slang or acronyms.

❑ If there is a potential for conflict, focus on the issue, not personalities.

❑ Stay at eye level with the persons to whom you are speaking.

❑ Maintain eye contact.

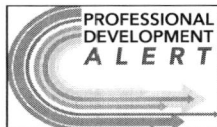

> **PROFESSIONAL DEVELOPMENT ALERT**
> Some issues, such as eye contact, have cultural implications. The principles in this chapter focus on American-style communication. Communication skills pertaining to culture may be found in Chapter 5.

❑ Avoid crossing your arms across your body. This indicates anger or avoidance.

❑ Listen actively. Don't send text messages or answer mobile phones when having a conversation with others. Look interested. Seek clarification if you don't understand what someone is saying. Invite them to seek clarification from you as well.

❏ Ask open-ended questions. Avoid asking questions that can be answered with a simple yes or no.

❏ Be aware of the personal space of others. This varies from person to person, but is usually no less than two to three feet.

❏ Avoid violating confidentiality on social networks such as Facebook.

❏ Avoid using all capital letters and be careful how you use exclamation points in writing. These can give the impression of anger.

The preceding skills are only a brief review. As noted, most of us, if asked, could recite these principles and add more.

Tips for Teaching Communication Skills

How can we be more creative when teaching others about communication? Here are some suggestions:

- Take learners by surprise. For example, suppose you are teaching in a classroom and speak inaudibly for a few minutes, or periodically pretend to send text messages when you should be listening to learners' questions. Use those examples to illustrate poor communication.

- Use role-play or skits to illustrate both good and poor communication.

- Design sample e-mails, text messages, and Facebook or Twitter postings and ask learners to identify how many good communication skills and how many poor communication skills they can find. Ask them to pay particular attention to violations of confidentiality.

- Ask learners to take a 10-minute walk through public areas of the organization and identify at least five good and five poor examples of communication. Be sure to tell them not to identify those they have observed; maintain confidentiality.

- Ask learners to think about their communication skills. Have them critique their skills by writing down examples of their communication during the past eight hours. This written critique is private and should not be shared in a classroom or other setting. It should be used almost as a journaling technique as learners write down their thoughts and feelings.

These are just a few ideas to get you started. Communication is one of the most important topics we can teach, but we need to be creative as to how we go about it!

31

Horizontal Violence: NPD's Role in Ending the Cycle

Horizontal violence (HV), sometimes referred to as horizontal bullying, is a well-known and, sadly, an all-too-common phenomenon among nurses. The International Council of Nurses defines HV as "behavior that humiliates, degrades, or otherwise indicates a lack of respect for the dignity and worth of an individual" (Dumont et al., 2012). Such behavior includes failure to intervene when a colleague is being bullied. A survey conducted by *Nursing2011* showed that the problem is quite prevalent, with 82% of respondents noting that they experienced or witnessed HV behaviors at least weekly or daily (Dumont et al., 2012).

What is the impact of the HV phenomenon? The following are some statistics compiled from research studies (Bartholomew, 2006; Dellasega, 2011):

- About 60% of newly registered nurses leave their first position within six months because of some form of HV.

- Verbal abuse contributes to 16% to 24% of staff nurse turnover and 25% to 42% of nurse administrator turnover.

- Fifty percent of people who experience HV continue to suffer from stress five years after the incident.

- Some studies show that nurses who experience HV take more than 50 sick days a year.

- Medication errors and other adverse occurrences are more likely to occur in an atmosphere of HV.

The preceding statistics show that HV takes a toll on the financial and emotional well-being of an organization and its employees. Nursing professional development (NPD) specialists play a critical role in reducing HV and its effects. Reduction involves administrative as well as education efforts.

Administrative

Sadly, administrators and nurse managers often ignore, hide, or even participate in HV. Excuses such as, "She may be a bully, but she's my best clinician," or "We can't take this too seriously, surviving bullying is a rite of passage" are all too common.

There must be consequences for committing or tacitly supporting HV. To stop this cycle NPD specialists must:

- Promote the development of and adherence to policies mandating zero tolerance for HV.

- Promote the development of and adherence to policies that allow grievances to be filed if HV occurs.

- Consequences of committing HV should be explicit, such as reprimands or comments noted on performance evaluations.

- Educate administrators and managers about the impact of HV by using objective statistics to show cost, adverse occurrences and errors, turnover, and emotional turmoil related to HV. It may very well be that organizational leaders are unaware of the cost, both emotional and financial, of HV and how it can impact patient care.

- Remind organizational leaders that nursing students are taught about HV in many nursing programs and how to deal with it, including filing grievances and, in some cases, lawsuits.

Staff Education

It is important that HV and its impact be part of ongoing education and training. Including it as part of annual mandatory training is recommended. Here are some more tips to make your HV training more dynamic:

- Include information about HV and how to deal with it as part of orientation. There may be some resistance to this idea. Many leaders and staff members refuse to look at HV as a problem; it's time they did.

- Include information about HV as part of preceptor training. As part of the education, include information about the rights of those being bullied (e.g., filing a grievance) and the impact it may have on the professional reputation of the person committing the bullying.

- Develop other means of HV education rather than simple lecture discussion. Incorporate role-play, dramatization, and simulated activities. If distance education is more practical, incorporate case studies, computer programs, or DVDs. Whenever possible incorporate some in-person activities. Actually participating in simulated activities helps nurses to practice dealing with bullying and, at times, helps bullies to recognize their own negative behaviors.

- Explain to all learners, administrators, managers, and staff members that bullying will not and cannot be tolerated. Staff nurses need to be taught how to respond to HV. For example, instead of silently accepting embarrassing remarks, they should be taught to confront the bully and note that "Those remarks are embarrassing and interfere with my ability to do my job."

It may not be possible to completely eliminate HV, but it is possible to reduce the frequency of occurrence and its negative consequences.

The Path to Stress-Free Nursing Professional Development

References

Bartholomew, K. (2006). *Ending Nurse-to-Nurse Hostility: Why Nurses Eat Their Young and Each Other.* Danvers, MA: HCPro, Inc.

Dellasega, C. (2011). *When Nurses Hurt Nurses.* Indianapolis, IN: STT.

Dumont, C., et al. (2012). Horizontal violence survey report. *Nursing 2011,* 42(1), 44-49.

Stagg, S. J., et al. (2011). Evaluation of a workplace bullying cognitive rehearsal program in a hospital setting. *The Journal of Continuing Education in Nursing,* 42(9), 395-403.

Nurturing the Professional Growth of the NPD Specialist

Learning Objectives

- Evaluate strategies to promote the professional growth and development of the NPD specialist.

- Initiate behaviors that enhance professional growth and development.

Section 3

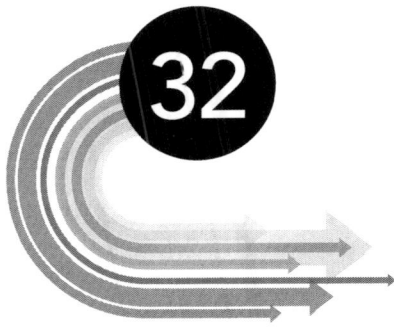

32 Nursing Professional Development Certification Test-Taking

Achieving nursing professional development (NPD) certification is a goal of many NPD specialists. In order to pass the certification exam, adequate preparation is necessary. It is essential to have a well thought-out study plan as soon as you decide you want to pursue certification. The first step is to start by determining eligibility.

Determining Eligibility

Begin by visiting the American Nurses Credentialing Center (ANCC) website (*www.nursecredentialing.org*). As of this writing, eligibility requirements are:

- *Hold a bachelor's or higher degree in nursing.*

- *Have practiced the equivalent of two years full-time as a registered nurse.*

- *Have a minimum of 4,000 hours of clinical practice in nursing professional development within the last five years. Hold a current, active RN license within a state or territory of the United States or the professional, legally recognized equivalent in another country.*

- *Have completed 30 hours of continuing education in nursing professional development within the last three years.[1]*

Preparing a Study Plan

After determining your eligibility, review the content outline and sample test questions available on the ANCC website. Review these items carefully, and objectively identify areas where you lack experience. These are the areas that will require significant focus as you prepare your study plan. The website also has a reference list that will help you to select good study resources.

---

[1]American Nurses Credentialing Center, Nursing Professional Development Certification Eligibility Criteria, *nursecredentialing.org/NPD-Eligibility.aspx.*

If you haven't already done so, identify your learning style (Avillion, 2010), which could be any of the following:

- **Visual learners:** Need to see what they are learning. They need to sit where they can see an instructor and prefer visual aids that contain color, illustrations, and graphics. Visual learners take copious notes and rely on notes as a study tool. They organize their notes carefully and depend on visual aids to learn.

- **Auditory learners:** Auditory learners prefer sounds to written words when studying. They don't care if they can see an instructor in a classroom as long as they can hear him or her. Auditory learners prefer auditory cues and too many illustrations, graphs, etc., in handouts and on PowerPoint® presentations are distracting to them. They talk through problems or study issues aloud and may prefer to have music playing in the background as they study.

- **Kinesthetic learners:** Kinesthetic learners learn by direct hands-on involvement. When studying they need frequent breaks to move around. They enjoy activities that allow them the freedom to move about, such as role-play and demonstration of psychomotor skills.

These are the three most commonly referred-to learning styles. There are subcategories of these learning styles, but this overview will hopefully help you determine your own learning preferences. Now, the next step is to come up with good study hygiene and to stick to it:

- Set up a specific time period to study. Adult learners have multiple family and career obligations. Explain to your family and friends that you are pursuing certification and work with them to establish your study routine. Schedule your study time just as you would any other important event (e.g., doctor's appointments, watching your children participate in sports events, etc.).

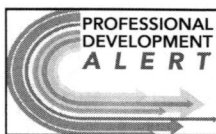

PROFESSIONAL DEVELOPMENT ALERT

Don't let anything except for true emergencies interfere with your study schedule. The first time you give in and take an extra carpool duty, or give up your study time to cook dinner even though it was your spouse's turn to do so, it will be assumed that your study time is arbitrary.

- Find a specific place to study. It needs to be your place and conducive to your particular learning style. It may be in a home office or at a local public or college library. If possible, don't share study space with family or friends during your study time. This will inevitably lead to distractions.

- Gather your study materials and keep them organized in your study place or in a book bag to take to your study place. Laptop, journal articles, books, etc., should be kept together. Don't scatter your study resources; you don't want to misplace any of them.

The Path to Stress-Free Nursing Professional Development

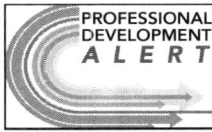

PROFESSIONAL
DEVELOPMENT
ALERT
Consider limiting the number of people you tell about taking the exam. This only increases the pressure on you to pass.

The Night Before and the Day of the Exam

The night before and day of the exam can be a bit nerve-racking; however, there are some strategies you can use to your advantage during this time. They include:

- ❑ Don't cram at the last minute. This will only increase your anxiety. Maintain a good study schedule and avoid cramming the night before and the day of the exam!

- ❑ The night before the exam, eat a good supper and get a good night's sleep. Avoid alcohol and foods and beverages that contain caffeine, which may interfere with your ability to sleep.

- ❑ Make sure to eat a good, healthy breakfast the morning of the exam, but don't overeat. A heavy meal may make you sleepy.

- ❑ You will receive confirmation of the date and time of the exam from the ANCC. Put these in your purse or pocket of the clothes you will be wearing so that you don't forget them. Also remember to bring photo identification with you.

- ❑ Make sure you know how to get to the designated test site. Arrive early. You don't want to get stuck in traffic or have a flat tire with only minutes to spare.

- ❑ Dress for comfort. Avoid your "skinny" jeans or tight shoes. It is important that you be as comfortable as possible.

- ❑ Wear a wristwatch. You will need to keep track of the time.

Tips for Taking Multiple-Choice Tests

Here are some tips for taking multiple-choice tests (Study Guides and Strategies, 2006).:

- ❑ Right before you begin your test, think positive thoughts. You have studied hard and you are prepared.

- ❑ Read all directions and listen to all instructions *attentively*!

- ❑ Multiple-choice questions consist of a question or an incomplete statement referred to as the "stem" of the question. The stem is followed by four choices, only one of which is the correct or best possible answer.

Read the stem and, without looking at the possible answers, come up with your own correct answer. Read the possible answers and see which one most closely matches your own correct answer.

❑ If you have trouble coming up with your own correct answer after first reading the stem, read the four choices and eliminate those that you know are incorrect. Then determine if the choices that are left are correct or incorrect by treating each one as a true/false statement and choose the one that is the mostly true.

❑ If two choices are quite similar, you can probably eliminate them, since there is only one correct answer.

❑ Eliminate choices that do not seem to fit grammatically with the stem or that are completely unfamiliar.

In summary, develop a good study action plan and stick to it. Good luck and happy studying!

Author's note: The author would like to acknowledge Kari L. Schmidt, MS, RN-BC, the director of employee and organizational development at Aurora Health Care in Milwaukee, and an expert in assisting NPD specialists to achieve certification in professional development. Schmidt is a past contributor to HCPro publications and has provided extensive background information on tips for passing the certification exam.

Reference

Avillion, A.E., et al (2010). *Innovation in Nursing Staff Development: Teaching Strategies to Enhance Learner Outcomes.* Danvers, MA: HCPro, Inc.

Study Guides and Strategies. (2006). Multiple choice tests. Retrieved February 5, 2012, from *www.studygs.net/tsttak3.htm.*

33 Submitting an Abstract for Presentation

As nursing professional development (NPD) specialists seek to advance in their chosen specialty, they are encouraged, and in some cases mandated, to prepare and submit abstracts for selection as a presenter at conferences and conventions. For some, the abstract submission process can be intimidating. For most of us it usually entails the challenge of explaining, in a few short written paragraphs, a concept that is dear to our role as educators. We must also convince those who review abstracts that ours is among the best!

Here are some tips for submitting an abstract:

- Identify the topic you would like to present. It needs to be something with which you are quite familiar and are very enthusiastic about. It also needs to have an innovative component. For example, orientation is a topic that appears at every professional development conference and convention almost without exception. Therefore, if you want to submit an abstract about orientation be sure you have something new and practical to offer. What is it about your orientation program that makes it particularly useful for other professional development colleagues? In other words, what is it about your presentation that makes it stand out from others on a similar topic?

- Identify the conference or convention for which you would like to be a presenter. If this is your first abstract submission, you may want to consider submitting to a smaller scale event rather than a national one. However, this is not a fixed rule. If you would like to aim for a national event, do so! Most conferences and conventions send out a call for abstract submission with instructions and perhaps a theme for that year's event. Explore the websites of event-sponsoring organizations and find one (or several) that seem to correlate with your topic.

- Nearly all abstract submissions are now completed online. Read all instructions carefully. Rather than write your initial submission online, write out a rough draft as a separate document first so that you have a chance to review it and think about its impact.

> **PROFESSIONAL DEVELOPMENT ALERT**
>
> Most conferences and conventions have options to present as a speaker or a poster pre-senter. Although poster presentations may seem easier for persons who are reluctant to speak in front of a large audience, posters have their own challenges. They need to tell your story relying primarily on visual aids. Many posters are quite sophisticated, so be prepared to compile a poster with an artistic flair. And, at some point, you will have to stand next to your poster and explain its contents as event attendees cluster around. Poster presentations are not easier than serving as a speaker, they are every bit as challenging!

- Ask a colleague to review your abstract prior to submitting it online. Preferably, this colleague will have successfully submitted abstracts and has experience as a poster presenter or speaker.

- Follow all directions carefully when submitting your abstract and be sure to adhere to any identified deadlines.

- Abstracts generally require that you identify your learning objectives, a brief content outline, and a paragraph or two that describes your topic. When writing your narrative paragraphs, start with a sentence that grabs attention. You will only have a limited number of words to convince the reviewers that your abstract should be selected. For instance, if your topic deals with orientation you might start by stating, "This presentation offers practical suggestions for decreasing the length of orientation while increasing retention and reducing turnover of newly hired nurses."

- If the submission guidelines permit, you may want to submit more than one abstract. Most major conferences and conventions receive a multitude of abstracts, so submitting more than one may increase your chances of acceptance.

- If accepted, you will receive instructions and deadlines for submission of handouts, PowerPoint® presentations, presenter biographies, etc. Be sure to complete and submit all required forms on time.

- If your abstract is not accepted, don't be discouraged! Submit your abstract to other events. Consider writing up your topic as a possible journal article. Never give up!

Following these tips will make submitting an abstract a little less stressful, and a little more successful.

34

Writing for Publication

Part of the professional growth and development of nursing professional development (NPD) specialists is mastering the art of writing for publication. Publication in the professional development field serves several purposes: It offers a chance for personal recognition for the writer, enhances departmental credibility within the organization, and adds to the unique body of knowledge that is NPD. The focus in this chapter is on writing an article for publication in a professional journal. Other opportunities for publication exist, including newsletters, contributing chapters to an edited book, or even writing a professional textbook; however, most initial formal efforts involve attempting to publish in a professional journal.

Publication is not an easy process. It takes perseverance, an ability to accept constructive criticism, and willingness to write and rewrite depending on editorial review.

Your first steps begin long before you write a single word. You can equate your steps to publication with the steps in planning and implementing an education program.

Assessment

A self-assessment is critical prior to writing. Why do you want to publish? What do you hope to achieve? What kinds of knowledge and skills do you have that, if published, will help colleagues in their own NPD practice? Here are some issues to address as part of your self assessment:

- Assess your own knowledge base. What is it you want to write about? An innovative education strategy? A project that shows how education affected job performance or patient outcomes? You need to select a topic with which you are very familiar and in which you have a passionate interest. Writing is a time-consuming process and generally involves editing, rewriting, and still more rewriting, so you need to be passionate about the topic and seeing your name in print.

- Determine if there is a need for the information you want to share. For example, you may have a passionate interest in identifying the various learning styles of adult learners, but is this interest enough to develop a publishable article? Editors are looking for articles or books that have a fresh, innovative approach. What is it about your approach to identifying learning styles that is unique? What new information do you have to share? It's not enough to rehash information that is already easily found in the current literature. You need to offer professional development colleagues information that is practical yet innovative. Think about what you would like to learn from published material on your topic of interest.

- Determine if you have the time and resources to devote to the publication process. Are you writing this article as part of your job responsibilities? If so, you should be able to use work time and resources to pursue publication. You will be enhancing your organization's reputation as well as your own when you publish and your place of employment is noted as part of your credentials. If you are writing this article on your own, you will need to plan for time to work on this endeavor at home. Make sure your family knows your plan and supports you in your publication efforts. They need to help you make the time you need to write.

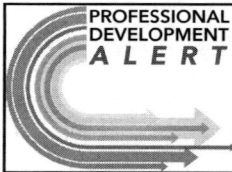

> **PROFESSIONAL DEVELOPMENT ALERT**
>
> If you are writing about a project you developed and implemented at work, be sure that you have your organization's approval to publish your findings. There may be political or other reasons why your administration may not want certain information available in the public arena.

Planning

After you've selected your topic, you are ready to move on to the planning stage. Just as it's important to plan the steps in the development of an education program, it's important to plan your writing strategy. Planning keeps you on track and saves time in the long run. The following are tips to plan your writing strategy:

- Decide if you will be writing alone or if you will have coauthors. If you are writing about a project that involved considerable time and effort from colleagues, it is probably a good idea to ask if they would like to participate in the writing process, or if they would be content with simply being acknowledged as having been instrumental to the project you are writing about. It may be politically advantageous to list as authors those who have helped with the project and are well-known or have publication experience. They may not contribute significantly to the actual writing process, but should still be included as an author.

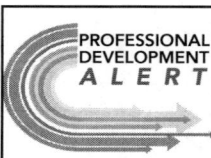

> **PROFESSIONAL DEVELOPMENT ALERT**
>
> Coauthoring articles can be both rewarding and frustrating. Matching writing styles and having all authors contributing equally to the process is a challenge. Writing alone means you don't have to deal with this problem, but also means you do not have assistance in the writing process. Weigh the benefits and disadvantages carefully.

- Write objectives for your article. What is it you want the readers to learn from your article? By identifying objectives, you will be able to better able focus your writing endeavors.

- Identify journals that fit with your topic. For instance, it may be appropriate to attempt to publish in a clinically-oriented journal if your project involves a teaching strategy that had a profound impact on clinical outcomes, but be aware that this type of choice mandates that the focus of your article must be the clinical aspects of the project. If you are more interested in the professional development aspects of your topic, then look for a journal that focuses on professional development and/or continuing education in nursing.

- Read the journals in which you hope to publish carefully. Observe the writing style and content of the articles. This will help you grasp the style that the journal approves for publication.

- Review the guidelines for authors from the journal(s) in which you hope to publish. Such guidelines are generally accessible on the journal's website or on the journal's publishing company's website. They are sometimes available in the journals themselves. Read the guidelines carefully and follow them meticulously. Most guidelines provide contact telephone numbers or e-mail addresses if you have questions. Don't hesitate to contact the journal for clarification about the guidelines. Most journal editors ask that you submit a letter of intent before you begin writing your article. This is to help the editor determine if your proposed article is suitable for the journal. Such a letter is extremely helpful and will save you time and effort if it turns out that your proposed article is not something that the editor believes is suitable for his or her journal.

- Avoid submitting the same article to several journals simultaneously. If it is accepted for publication by more than one journal you will then have to choose which journal you prefer. This is not a professional approach to writing. Submit your article to one journal at a time.

PROFESSIONAL DEVELOPMENT ALERT

Once a journal accepts your article and publishes it, the publishing company, not you, holds the copyright to that article. This means you cannot reprint or distribute copies of the article without the permission of the publisher. Also, you cannot submit the same article for publication in other journals. You can write a new article for submission elsewhere on the same topic, but not the identical article that has already been published. Note that the article must be significantly different (alter the focus, change the objectives) to avoid violating copyright regulations.

Implementation

Now you get to start writing! Remember that you will write and rewrite your manuscript as you respond to constructive criticism from trusted colleagues and journal editors. The following are some tips to keep in mind as you being the actual writing process:

- Compose an outline that is based on your identified objectives or goals for that article. An outline keeps you focused and helps to ensure that you meet the objectives you identified.

- Begin with a short introductory paragraph that grabs readers' attention. A first sentence that says something like, "The blended orientation program developed and implemented by the professional development department at X Hospital had a significant impact on reducing turnover and increasing retention" will surely trigger interest.

- Be clear and concise in your writing. Avoid making broad generalizations. Remember, the reader is not familiar with what you have accomplished. You need to explain what you did, why you did it, and the results of your actions.

- Be sure to reference your work meticulously. It is a scholarly work and must be appropriately referenced. The author guidelines will tell you which reference style to use.

Evaluation

Going through the evaluation process can trigger feelings of both euphoria and discouragement. Positive comments are always a boost to the ego; however, all writers must respond to the constructive criticism they receive from editors of journals. Don't take criticism personally. A thorough evaluation will only help you to improve your manuscript. Keep in mind to:

- Ask for help. Ask a professional development colleague who has publication experience to critique your article before submitting it for publication. Ideally, this should be someone from outside your organization who has no knowledge of the particular project you are writing about. This way he or she can help to point out areas that are unclear or ambiguous. Someone from within the organization may be too familiar with your topic and "fill in the blanks" without asking for appropriate clarification. Just as ideally, the colleague should not be a close friend, but a professional colleague who will offer objective constructive criticism without fear of offending you.

- Expect edits. Articles submitted to professional journals are generally blind reviewed (i.e., the reviewers will not know who you are or your place of employment) by at least two reviewers. They and the editor will make comments that usually include requests for revision. Do not be offended by the need to rewrite. It is almost unheard of for an article to be accepted without some type of revision being mandated. Review the editorial comments and address them carefully. Don't hesitate to seek clarification if you do not understand what is being asked of you.

- Don't give up! Even if your article is not accepted for publication, you will learn a great deal about the publication process. Absorb constructive criticism, and continue to write and pursue publication.

When writing for publication, from formulating an idea to seeing your article in print, you will have times of excitement and frustration. There will be rewrites to do, questions to answer, and points to clarify. Just remember that any struggles are well worth the joy of seeing your ideas in print.

35

Grant Writing

By Barbara A. Brunt, MA, MN, RN-BC, NE-BC

The first step in the process of writing a grant is researching grantors. Where do you go to find out about grants? First, look in your organization's historical files for grant opportunities that slipped away, and examine similar organizations' websites, newsletters, and annual reports for notations about grants received. Consider corporations and foundations in your local area. Talk with others who have been successful getting grants about possible opportunities. There are many online databases that list available grants—some of these sites are listed in the suggested readings at the end of this chapter.

Grants that are available to health professionals primarily fall into six categories: foundation grants, hospital-based grants, professional association grants, corporate partnerships, pre- and post-doctoral fellowships, and federal grants.

Most grant proposals have common elements: executive summary or abstract, project description or statement of need/problem, design/methodology section (including instruments), budget and timetable, organization information and/or biosketch of primary investigator, conclusion, and letters of support. For a chart on types of grants, see Figure 35.1 (at *www.hcpro.com/downloads/10170*).

Before starting to write, make sure you do the following:

- Review the literature and successfully funded proposals from the same funding agency

- Talk with experts in the field

- Obtain consultation as necessary

- Identify a relevant question that would be of interest to the funding source

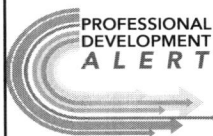

Be informed—you need to tie in with the goal of the funding source. To do that you can read the annual report or check the website, use the contact person listed on the application as a resource or find a mentor, and be very aware of deadlines. Creating a realistic time frame up front can save headaches on the back end. Estimate how long it will take you to complete the application and then double that time. Preliminary development should start six to eight months prior to the application deadline.

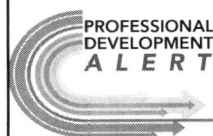

PROFESSIONAL DEVELOPMENT ALERT

Before starting to write you need to focus on quality, not quantity. Network and talk with colleagues who have been through the process. It may be helpful to use a team approach and recruit others based on their interest and expertise. It is important to make sure you have enough time to work on this—schedule time for grant writing just as you schedule time for vacations and other projects.

PROFESSIONAL DEVELOPMENT ALERT

Three characteristics of a good grant proposal are: (1) meaningful question—is it important to the funding agency and consistent with its mission and goals? (2) good science—does it reflect thorough planning and the state of the science in the proposed area of study? (3) careful application techniques—does the proposal comply with all instructions, is it neat, logical, and complete?

When you start writing your grant application, follow the directions explicitly! Failure to include necessary information or going beyond the required word limit can result in automatic rejection. Use key words and objectives from the application packet. Once you think the application is perfect, give it to several others to review. Have someone with experience writing grants review it, as well as someone with a good ability to proofread and edit. Make sure you match your request to the award range, and include graphics to give the proposal visual pizzazz.

Once you submit the proposal, the waiting begins. Most proposals indicate when feedback will be given. If it goes beyond that date, feel free to call or write and ask for an update. Don't be discouraged if your study does not get funded. Generally there are limited resources so even well written studies get rejected.

Survival tips for grant writing include the following:

- ❏ Find a mentor with research experience

- ❏ Join forces with other organizations/groups to apply for grants

- ❏ Write, rewrite, proof, re-proof, and include colleagues in reading drafts

- ❏ Break the project into manageable pieces and strictly follow grant deadlines

- ❏ Be sure to include all institutional review approvals for a research grant

❑ Read proposal for clarity, organization, ease of understanding, and correct grammar

❑ Be flexible and open to feedback and suggestions

❑ Remember the five critical qualities the writer must possess, the "5 P's:" passion, planning, persuasion, persistence, and patience.

Once you receive a grant, you need to manage it. Set up mechanisms for oversight of the project, and follow the guidelines from the agency for reports. Make sure you have enough time to achieve the project goals, and ensure you have enough time to complete the work needed. And of course, make a plan to disseminate your findings.

Suggested Readings

Browning, B. A. (2011). *Grant Writing for Dummies*. 4th Ed. Hoboken, NJ: John Wiley & Sons.

Holtzclaw, B. J., Kenner, C., and Walden, M. (2009). *Grant Writing Handbook for Nurses*. 2nd Ed. Sudbury, MA: Jones and Bartlett.

Johnson, V. M. (2011). *Grant Writing 101: Everything You Need to Start Raising Funds Today*. New York: McGraw-Hill.

Melnyk, B. M. & Fineout-Overholt, E. (2011). Writing a successful grant proposal to fund research and evidence-based practice implementation projects. In B.M. Melnyk and E. Fineout-Overholt. *Evidence-based Practice in Nursing and Healthcare: A Guide to Best Practice*. (pp. 449-473). 2nd Ed. Philadelphia: Wolters Kluwer Health.

Online Resources

www.Grantwhisperer.com
www.Foundationcenter.org
www.Grants.gov
www.Foundationcenter.org/getstarted/learnabout/proposalwriting.html
www.fundsnetservices.com

36

Nursing Professional Development Research

Nursing professional development (NPD) research is essential for several reasons:

- NPD research is a foundation of evidence-based practice.

- NPD research adds to the body of knowledge of nursing in general and NPD in particular.

- NPD research enhances the credibility of the specialty and the recognition of its practitioners.

The formal research process is conducted scientifically and under the guidance/direction of one who is trained and educated in the research process. Some NPD specialists, educated at the doctoral level, may possess this type of education. However, given the rather small number of NPD specialists currently prepared at the doctoral level, it is arguably more likely that many of us look to collaborate with nurse researchers when formalizing NPD research. NPD specialists who work in large teaching facilities may have easier access to resources for this collaboration compared to those who work in smaller facilities. However, there are resources available to all if we know where to look. The following are some practical suggestions for conducting formal NPD research.

Research Topic

All research begins with a question and an idea. How will changing a particular education program from classroom to blended learning affect job performance and patient outcomes? If you revise and expand the preceptor program, will that have a positive impact on retention? How would an increase in emergency simulation drills impact patient outcomes during actual emergencies?

What questions do you have? What would you like to know about the impact of education on job performance, patient outcomes, and organizational effectiveness? You probably have lots of ideas about how you would like to demonstrate the value of education. These are the ideas and questions you will bring with you when you work with your research experts. You will also bring with you any initial research you may have conducted relying on evaluation data that demonstrate a link between education and knowledge acquisition, behavior, results, and return on investment (ROI). Now you need to identify researchers with whom to work.

Identifying Research Colleagues

Your first step is to review the policies and guidelines pertaining to research within your organization. There is an institutional review board (IRB) that reviews and approves research proposals, oversees their implementation, and reviews outcomes at any facility that allows research within its walls. Review the policies and guidelines carefully. Find out what is required of you as a researcher.

Next, if you are fortunate enough to have a nurse researcher as an employee of your organization, set up a meeting with him or her. If you don't have a nurse researcher, here are some ideas of how to go about finding one:

- Talk to faculty members who supervise nursing students within your organization. Many of them either have research experience or are working on graduate degrees that require research. They may be glad of the opportunity to collaborate with you or they may know someone who would be.

- If you don't have nursing student affiliations, contact the nearest university or college that has a nursing program. Faculty and students are often looking for collaborative research opportunities.

- Sigma Theta Tau International Honor Society of Nursing (*www.nursingsociety.org*) is an excellent resource. Their website lists affiliations and contact information. You will probably have success collaborating with members of this society.

- Consider collaborating with colleagues from other healthcare facilities within your geographic region. Pool your resources and work with other NPD specialists.

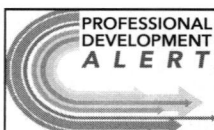

> **PROFESSIONAL DEVELOPMENT ALERT**
>
> Before talking to colleagues who are not directly employed by your organization (and that includes faculty from student affiliations) check with your manager or director. There may be political considerations of which you are unaware.

- Be prepared to reward the hard work of those with whom you collaborate. If you want to publish the results of your research, your colleagues should be invited to participate in the writing process. If you plan on presenting the results at a conference or convention, your colleagues should be invited to be copresenters. At the very least, if they decline the opportunity to publish or present, they need to be acknowledged as being instrumental in the process.

Some Tips on What to Expect

Research is not a quick process. It is exciting but requires extensive preparation and detailed implementation. When choosing someone with whom to collaborate, choose wisely. You need to respect the researcher and be willing to accept his or her constructive criticism.

After listening to your ideas, the researcher will help you to narrow your focus and clarify your research question. For example, think about the example of the impact of increasing emergency simulation drills. The researcher will ask questions such as:

- What population of nurses are you going to include in your study? Critical care nurses? Staff nurses? Which units are you going to include? Are you including only RNs in your study or did you want to include LPNs and/or nursing assistants as well?

- Why have you chosen this particular group of nurses? Are you interested in finding out if additional education enhances the performance of noncritical care nurses in an emergency? Or are you focusing on nurses new to critical care?

- How are you going to measure enhanced performance? How are you going to compare before and after performance? Who will assess performance?

- What dangers does this study pose to patients, families, and/or staff members? How will you control those dangers?

- What will you do with the results from your study? How will you share them with the IRB? How will you use the results to improve job performance and patient care?

The preceding questions are just some of many that you will need to address. As you clarify the research question and the focus, you and your research colleague(s) will need to determine what statistical analysis will be used. You'll need to conduct a literature review to support your research question and the design of your study. You will also need to write a detailed proposal to present to your IRB and an oral defense of what you want to do and why.

Even as you begin to implement your study, you may find that unexpected obstacles arise. You and your research expert will try to identify these obstacles beforehand, but will also need to be prepared to deal with the unexpected. You will need to evaluate your data and be prepared for unexpected results. For example, how will you deal with results that show education did not have a positive impact on job performance?

These ideas and suggestions are just a jumping off spot for you as you begin to think about designing and implementing a research project. Remember that research is essential to enhancing the credibility of our specialty and important to the identification of education strategies that improve job performance and enhance patient outcomes.

37

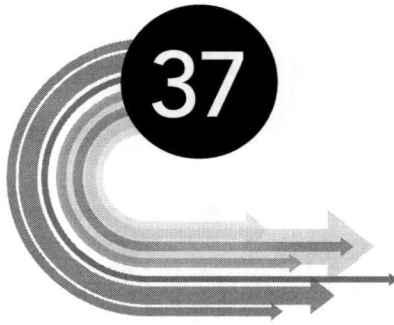

Career Advancement for NPD Specialists

Author's note: The levels of expertise for nursing professional development (NPD) specialists are more fully explained in Chapter 38, Identifying Levels of Expertise of NPD Specialists. This chapter focuses on suggestions for career advancement (career ladder).

Although significant attention has been given to developing career advancement programs for staff nurses, such as clinical ladders, little attention has been paid to developing similar programs for NPD specialists. The following suggestions for career advancement are based on Benner's (1984) levels of expertise and adapted by Avillion (2011) for the NPD field.

Career Advancement Action Plan for the Novice

Novices are not NPD specialists. They are RNs who have demonstrated an interest in and aptitude for providing education and training as evidenced by their work as preceptors and/or helping to train and educate their peers and subordinates. The following are some actions for the novices to take as they pursue their career advancement:

- Obtain BSN (if not already baccalaureate prepared)

- Complete preceptor training and function as preceptor

- Identify pursuit of teaching opportunities as part of goals during annual performance evaluation

- Assist unit-based nurse educator or NPD specialist (whichever is applicable for your organization) with in-service training

- Assist unit-based nurse educator or NPD specialist (whichever is applicable for your organization) with education needs assessment and facets of continuing education

- Pursue continuing education that focuses on adult education and professional development

- Seek out an NPD mentor

Career Advancement Action Plan for Advanced Beginners

Advanced beginners do not meet the definition of an NPD specialist according to the Nursing Professional Development Scope and Standards of Practice (ANA/NNSDO, 2010), which states that the NPD specialist is a licensed RN with a graduate degree. If the graduate degree is in a related discipline, then the baccalaureate degree must be in nursing. The advanced beginner does not have a graduate degree, and functions as a unit-based educator. Examples of career advancement action plan statements for the advanced beginner who wants to pursue the role of NPD specialist include:

- Identify a graduate degree program with a major in a field that will help in the advancement to NPD specialist. Examples include nursing, adult education, and organizational development.

- Enroll in an appropriate graduate degree program.

- Identify a target date for completion of graduate degree.

- Actively assist the NPD specialist with activities that go beyond the unit-based in-service and assisting with unit-based continuing education. Participate in analyzing education needs for the organization and seek out opportunities to become involved in housewide continuing education efforts.

- Consult resources such as *The Journal for Nurses in Staff Development* and *The Journal of Continuing Education in Nursing* as well as books that focus on adult education and professional development. Apply information learned to own practice.

- Pursue continuing education in the field of adult education and professional development.

- Actively assist with reaction, learning, and behavioral levels of evaluation.

- Pursue continuing education pertaining to evidence-based practice (EBP) in professional development.

- Identify a NPD mentor and work on developing career goals with him or her.

- Identify pursuit of a graduate degree as a career goal during annual performance evaluation.

- Identify goals specific to the pursuit of the NPD role during annual performance evaluation.

Career Advancement Action Plan for Competent NPD Specialists

The competent NPD specialist is prepared at the graduate level and has a minimum of two to three years of NPD experience. Their biggest challenges involve looking at the long-range effects of their education efforts. They may react too quickly to challenges rather than stop and gather evidence to justify their actions. Competents need to focus on the intricacies of program evaluation and developing an EBP foundation.

Here are some examples of action plan statements for career advancement:

- Pursue professional development continuing education with a focus on EBP in professional development and assessing the impact of education on job performance and patient outcomes.

- Work with a mentor who will help to facilitate professional development goals and aspirations.

- Work with a proficient and/or expert NPD specialist to gather and analyze evidence pertaining to the impact of education on job performance and patient outcomes.

- Pursue NPD certification.

- Consider pursuing additional graduate level courses. Determine if a doctorate degree is part of career goals.

- Join professional associations at regional and national levels such as the National Nursing Staff Development Organization (*www.nnsdo.org*) and The American Society for Training and Development (*www.astd.org*).

- Pursue membership in housewide educational committees such as risk management and begin to assume responsibility for significant committee tasks.

- Under the guidance of a mentor and/or proficient and expert NPD specialists, collaborate on writing an abstract or an article for publication in a professional journal.

- Earn a minimum of 10 contact hours annually in continuing education that focuses on staff development.

Career Advancement Action Plan for Proficient NPD Specialists

The proficient NPD specialist has a minimum of five years of experience and sees situations as a whole rather than as individual components. He or she is usually certified in NPD and begins to assume more leadership responsibilities.

The following are some examples of career action plan statements for the proficient NPD:

- Demonstrate sophisticated implementation of EBP in professional development.

- Assume chairpersonship of organizational committees as appropriate.

- Gather and analyze evidence pertaining to education needs and knowledge gaps from committees.

- Enhance ability to perform results evaluation and document the impact of education on job performance and patient outcomes.

- Is an active member of professional associations. Serve on association committees and task forces.

- Submit abstracts for presentation at conferences and conventions.

- Submit article(s) for publication in professional journals.

- Continue to work with a mentor to work on professional goals.

- Act as a mentor for less experienced colleagues.

- Earn a minimum of 15 hours of continuing education focused on professional development, particularly on sophisticated evaluation methods and leadership qualities.

Career Advancement Action Plan for Expert NPD Specialists

An expert NPD specialist has a minimum of 10 years of NPD experience. The expert NPD possesses a doctorate degree and focuses on sophisticated levels of NPD practice.

Examples of career action statements for the expert include the following:

- Chair committees at the organizational level

- Actively serve as a mentor for persons within and outside of the organization

- Run for office of professional associations

- Present papers at local and national conferences and conventions

- Publish articles pertaining to the impact of education on job performance and patient outcomes

- Budget for professional development endeavors

- Initiate and participate in professional development research

- Seek out leadership opportunities

References

ANA/NNSDO. (2010). *Nursing Professional Development Scope and Standards of Practice*. Silver Spring, MD: Authors.

Avillion, A. E. (2011). *Professional Growth in Staff Development: Strategies for New and Experienced Educators*. Danvers, MA: HCPro, Inc.

Benner, P. (1984). *From Novice to Expert: Excellence and Power in Clinical Nursing Practice*. Menlo Park, CA: Addison-Wesley Publishing Company.

Administrative Issues

Learning Objectives

- Explain the impact of NPD administrative issues on NPD practice.

- Identify ways to meet NPD administrative practice needs.

Section 4

38

Identifying Levels of Expertise of NPD Specialists

To date, minimal time has been spent in identifying levels of expertise specific to nursing professional development (NPD) specialists. NPD specialists are the go-to source for facilitating career advancement programs (e.g., clinical ladders) for staff nurses and promoting the professional growth and development of our clinical colleagues. However, little attention has been devoted to identifying levels of expertise for NPD specialists or nurturing their professional growth (see Chapter 37, Career Advancement for NPD Specialists).

Here are some suggestions to help guide you as you identify levels of NPD expertise for the purpose of developing not only career advancement programs, but job descriptions and competencies as well (Avillion, 2011). The chart in Figure 38.1, "Overview of Professional Development Levels of Expertise" summarizes these levels (visit *www.hcpro.com/downloads/10170*).

Novice

The novice has no experience as an NPD specialist. Novices are staff nurses who demonstrate a talent for education as they help their colleagues to function in a new situation, work with orientees, function as preceptors, provide patient education, etc. Novices express an interest in the education process and seek out opportunities to work with unit-based educators or NPD specialists.

Novices have no formal training or education in professional development or related fields. Therefore, it is suggested that they be encouraged to learn more about the specialty of professional development in theory as well as in practice. Books and journals devoted to professional development should be on their professional reading list. They should be trained as preceptors and introduced to the education process by helping with just-in-time training and in-service. Most of all, we need to make time to sit down with novices and talk about what being a unit-based educator or NPD specialist entails. We should also talk to novices' managers and ask if they have indicated their interest in pursuing or expanding their roles as staff nurses to include more education responsibilities.

PROFESSIONAL
DEVELOPMENT
A L E R T

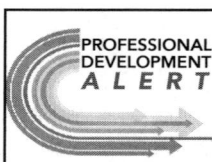

Include discussions with nurse managers as you identify Novices. Unless managers are included in encouraging the development of Novices, they may become resentful of the time Novices spend devoted to education activities. Managers may even accuse you of trying to stead members of their staff and take them away from direct patient care.

Advanced Beginners

Advanced beginners are not NPD specialists. They generally function as unit-based educators with a focus on in-service and assist the NPD specialist with more sophisticated aspects of education. Advanced beginners have dealt with enough real-life education situations on the unit level to identify basic components of the education process. They possess a BSN in nursing and have received some training and education with emphasis on the principles of adult education. They may hold a dual role consisting of staff nurse responsibilities as well as education responsibilities.

Advanced beginners are of great support to the NPD specialists. They can participate in data gathering and help with evaluation of education. However, their focus is primarily on unit-based activities. They assist with the development of continuing education, but based on their level of education and training, are not able to independently initiate a thorough analysis of evaluation data nor can they design continuing education independently.

If advanced beginners are interested in pursuing the role of NPD specialist, they must have a plan for obtaining a graduate degree and obtaining education specific to the role of an adult educator; however, don't discount the role of advanced beginners as unit-based educators. You may choose to have this as an ongoing role, particularly in larger healthcare organizations. People who choose to remain in the role are valuable resources and should be encouraged to progress in their unit-based activities.

Competents

Competents are NPD specialists, educated at the graduate level. According to the Nursing Professional Development Scope and Standards of Practice (ANA/NNSDO, 2010), NPD specialists are licensed RNs with a graduate degree. If the graduate degree is in a related discipline, then the baccalaureate degree must be in nursing. They have been in the role for at least two to three years and are able to independently carry out basic needs assessment and plan and implement in-service and simple continuing education programs.

Competents need help to evaluate program data and translate such data into professional development evidence-based practice. They are valuable committee members, but need help translating committee data into useful professional development evidence. They are not yet ready to assume significant leadership roles, such as chairpersons of committees. Continuing education should include ways to acquire and expand leadership skills.

Competents do not have the speed or flexibility of the proficient or expert NPD specialist. They still look at the parts of an education program rather than seeing situations as a whole. For example, they are still likely to overreact to a few negative program evaluation comments rather than perform a complete analysis of available data. Their continuing education should include information on more sophisticated ways to analyze data and assess the impact of education on patient outcomes and job performance.

Proficients

Proficients have a minimum of five years of experience and are able to perceive situations as "wholes" rather than in "parts." They are able to serve as mentors and can assume the role of committee chairpersons. They generally hold NPD certification.

Proficients think, speak, and react in terms of evidence-based NPD practice. They rely on evidence to guide their decision-making and are always pursuing evidence pertaining to the impact of education on job performance and patient outcomes.

> **PROFESSIONAL DEVELOPMENT ALERT**
>
> Proficients may be among the most difficult NPD specialists to retain. They have enough experience that they may become bored with the day-to-day operations of NPD. They need support and opportunities to grow professionally, such as enhanced leadership roles, working on NPD research, and opportunities to present and publish.

Experts

Experts have a minimum of 10 years experience in the NPD field. They function on an intuitive, instinctive level and can quickly grasp the essentials of any professional development situation. Often prepared at the doctorate level, experts usually occupy leadership positions like directors of the NPD department and/or are significantly involved in NPD research efforts.

Experts often feel that they have "seen and done it all" and are prone to burnout. Like proficients, experts need to be nurtured and provided with opportunities for new and varied experiences. These often take the form of promoting NPD research and adding to the NPD body of knowledge.

References

ANA/NNSDC. (2010). *Nursing Professional Development Scope and Standards of Practice*. Silver Spring, MD: Authors.

Avillion, A. E. (2011). *Professional Growth in Staff Development: Strategies for New and Experienced Educators*. Danvers, MA: HCPro, Inc.

39

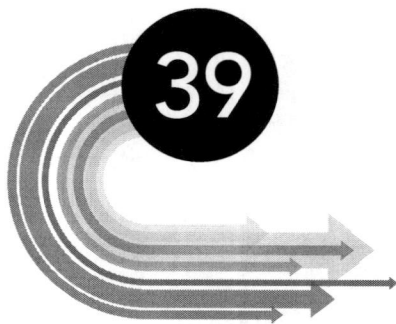

Measuring the Impact of Education: Nursing Professional Development Evidence-Based Practice

Evidence-based practice (EBP) in nursing professional development (NPD) is the process of relying on evidence to identify best practices, evaluate and revise education and training, and determine the need for new education endeavors. Critical to all EBP in NPD is the ability to gather and analyze data to show the impact of education on job performance, patient outcomes, and organizational effectiveness.

The purpose of all levels of evaluation is to gather and analyze data and to use that analysis to improve education services. The overall goal of NPD is to offer education that has a positive impact on job performance and patient outcomes. All aspects of our practice should be driven by this overall goal. It is not possible to measure education's impact unless we have a practice that is grounded in evidence. It is also impossible to have a credible department without providing evidence of education's positive impact on organizational effectiveness (Avillion, 2011).

Let's look at the five levels of evaluation as they relate to EBP (Avillion, 2011).

Reaction

Reaction data measures learner satisfaction with the education experience and the environment in which it was provided. These types of data can be used as a building block of evidence. Suppose you are advocating for improvements to classrooms that are cold and have poor acoustics. Learners complain about the cold or having trouble hearing instructors. These kinds of concerns should be looked at not merely as, "We need warmer classrooms," or "Instructors just have to speak up." Instead, look at higher levels of evaluation. Is the environment having a negative impact on learning or behaviors? In other words, is the environment impeding learning? This kind of correlation with reaction and higher levels of evaluation can provide evidence to help you improve learning environments.

Learning

Learning, usually measured as part of a post-test or skills demonstration, is generally limited to the immediate learning environment. It is often used in situations such as CPR certification or learning to master a new piece of patient care equipment in an in-service situation.

Data from learning can be used in conjunction with reactive data, as shown in the previous discussion regarding reactive data. Learning is often a prerequisite for skills like transferring new knowledge or skill from the learning environment to the actual work setting. Demonstrating learning can be a fearful experience, especially if demonstrated learning (e.g., skill acquisition or Advanced Cardiac Life Support certification) is necessary to maintain one's job or apply for career advancement. Learning is part of the evidence necessary before a nurse can fulfill certain job responsibilities, such as successfully completing a competency-based orientation.

Learning must also be used as a prior step to behavior, results, and return on investment (ROI) levels of evaluation. For example, did learning take place according to established criteria and learning objectives? If so, we can look at how that learning was applied (or not applied) in the work setting.

It is not enough to simply provide evidence that learning occurred. A nurse may obtain CPR certification without difficulty (meaning learning took place), but if he or she fails to perform CPR accurately in the actual work setting, knowledge is insufficient. Therefore, we need evidence of desired behaviors.

Behavior

Behavior is the correct application of knowledge gained in the actual work setting. We need to provide evidence as to how learning has influenced work-related behaviors. An education program on the legal aspects of documentation can only be judged a success if the nurses who attended the program apply their knowledge as evidenced by a review of documentation. A comparison of pre- and post-education documentation can provide evidence that there was an improvement in adherence to legal guidelines of nursing documentation. This is the type of report you want to provide to nursing managers. They want to know that the time nurses spent participating in education (and away from patient care) was worthwhile. Only if you take the time to evaluate behavior can you provide them with the evidence that it did.

Practicing in this type of EBP manner allows you to communicate effectively. When faced with challenging questions about the usefulness of educational activities, you need to be able to have this type of evidence readily available.

Behavior is not enough, however. Certainly it can provide impressive evidence about the usefulness of education. But the true impact of education (and the credibility of your department) is best demonstrated by results evaluative data.

Results (Impact)

Results, quite simply, are the assessment of the impact of education on job performance and patient outcomes. Behavior evidence, such as in the preceding example of legalities of documentation, may be sufficient. Results would be indicated if documentation was reviewed in a court of law and found to provide evidence of appropriate patient care. Hopefully, such an example is a rare occurrence. But in many cases, results must be assessed.

For example, suppose you have determined that a knowledge gap exists regarding appropriate care of the patient with an indwelling catheter. Nosocomial urinary tract infections in that particular patient population have increased throughout the nursing units. Your department provides a detailed education program not only on the care of the patient but on the importance of hand washing and intervening when other healthcare providers fail to wash their hands. The program takes time, money, and effort on the part of the NPD specialists and the members of the nursing staff who must attend the program. You need to show not only evidence of learning and behavior but of impact or results as well. You need to show that after education was provided, the rate of infections decreased. This is objective evidence that education made a difference.

Return on Investment

Return on investment (ROI) is generally conducted on programs that have significant organizational impact and require a significant amount of money to plan, implement, and evaluate. ROI requires that you measure the expense of a program compared to profit or significant impact. For example, suppose you revise both the preceptor and nursing orientation programs. You believe that such revisions will reduce turnover and increase retention as well as save the organization money.

To provide evidence of results as well as ROI, you need to work with human resources to gather data pertaining to recruitment, retention, and turnover. You also need to work with the financial office to determine the cost of these items. By comparing such data before and after program revisions, you can show monetary impact as well as results. You could provide evidence of the rate of increase in retention, decrease in turnover, and the money saved by these results.

In summary, you need to have the evidence that NPD enhances organizational effectiveness. You can only do this by identifying evidence and objectively communicating that evidence to administration, management, and staff.

Reference

Avillion, A. E. (2011). *The Survival of Staff Development: Measure Outcomes and Demonstrate Value to Establish an Indispensable Department*. Danvers, MA: HCPro, Inc.

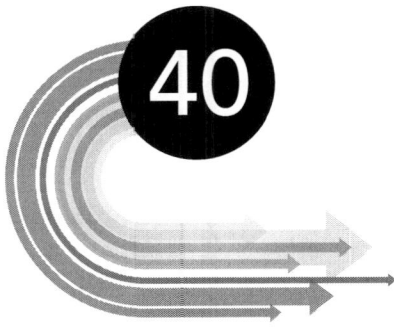

40   Job Description Statements

Author's note: These sample job description statements are based on Chapter 38, Identifying Levels of Expertise of NPD Specialists.

All organizations have their own templates for job descriptions. Basic information such as education and experience requirements, physical requirements, etc., are included. The focus of this chapter is on sample job description statements specific to nursing professional development (NPD). These statements are grounded in the standards identified in the Nursing Professional Development Scope and Standards of Practice (ANA/NNSDO, 2010) as adapted by Avillion (2011).

Novices

Novices are not part of the NPD department. These are generally staff nurses who have been identified by members of the NPD department and/or nurse managers as people who have the potential to pursue the role of unit-based educator or NPD specialist. Therefore, NPD job description statements are not available. The NPD emphasis for novices is identifying likely candidates and nurturing their professional growth as identified in Chapter 38.

Advanced Beginners

Recall that advanced beginners are prepared at the baccalaureate level and are not NPD specialists, but generally fill the role of unit-based educator. Therefore, you will notice that most of the sample statements include the word "assist" in their foundations.

Here are some sample job description statements:

- Plans and implements in-service education for designated unit(s).

- Assists the NPD specialist with the design of unit-based needs assessments and collection of needs assessment data.

- Assists the NPD specialist with planning and implementing unit-specific continuing education.

- Assists the NPD specialist to gather program evaluation data.

- Assists the NPD specialist with program evaluation analysis.

- Works with nurse managers of designated unit(s) to identify in-service needs.

- Works with the preceptors of designated unit(s) to facilitate preceptor effectiveness.

- Attends staff meetings of designated unit(s).

- Attends NPD department staff meetings and works with other members of the NPD department to promote the professional growth and development of the members of the nursing department.

Competents

Competents have two to three years of experience as NPD specialists. You will notice that some statements acknowledge that experience and others show areas in which competents need assistance and guidance. The following are some examples of competent job description statements:

- Plans, designs, and implements in-service and continuing education based on needs assessment data and incorporating the principles of adult education.

- Uses a variety of teaching strategies and audiovisuals to facilitate achievement of program objectives.

- In collaboration with NPD colleagues, designs needs assessments and collects needs assessment data.

- Gathers and analyzes evidence pertaining to reaction, learning, and behavioral levels of evaluation.

- Involves learners in needs assessments and identification of learning objectives.

- Serves as a member of designated nursing and organizational committees.

- Gathers evidence pertaining to education needs and activities from committees and assists in analyzing that evidence.

- Works with staff, managers, and administration to identify learning needs and implement appropriate education.

- Attends professional development department staff meetings and works with other members of the department to promote the professional growth and development of the employees of the organization.

Proficients

Proficients are experienced NPD specialists. Their job description statements show a more advanced level of practice and independence compared to competents:

- Plans, designs, and implements all types of education independently.

- Coordinates and manages complex educational offerings based on organizational goals and objectives.

- Uses and develops a variety of innovative teaching strategies and audiovisuals to facilitate the achievement of program objectives.

- Designs needs assessments and uses data from these assessments as part of evidence-based practice (EBP) in professional development.

- Gathers and analyzes evidence pertaining to reaction, learning, behavior, impact, and return on investment levels of evaluation.

- Involves learners in needs assessments and identification of learning objectives.

- Serves as a member of designated nursing and organizational committees and serves as chair as appropriate.

- Gathers evidence pertaining to education needs and activities from committees and analyzes that evidence.

- Works with staff, managers, and administration to identify learning needs and implement appropriate education. Implements EBP in professional development in all NPD activities.

- Is an active member of professional associations.

- Submits abstracts for presentation at local and national conferences and conventions.

- Submits articles for publication in professional journals.

- Attends professional development department staff meetings and works with other members of the department to promote the professional growth and development of the employees of the organization.

- Assumes the role of mentor for less experienced professional development colleagues.

Experts

Experts are the most sophisticated of NPD practitioners. Job description statements should reflect that sophistication. Examples include:

- Responsible for coordinating all aspects of education for the NPD department based on organizational goals, objectives, and priorities.

- Ensures that the most current and innovative teaching strategies are used to meet learner needs and provide quality education.

- Ensures that all five levels of evaluation are implemented as appropriate.

- Ensures that EBP in professional development is the foundation of all NPD activities.

- Chairs committees at the organizational level.

- Analyzes data from committees and applies them to EBP in professional development.

- Works with staff, managers, and administration to identify learning needs and implement appropriate education.

- Actively participates in professional associations, demonstrated by seeking office or committee appointments at the national level.

- Presents papers at national conferences and conventions that focus on professional development.

- Publishes articles pertaining to professional development in professional journals.

- Conducts NPD department meetings.

- Budgets for NPD activities.

- Initiates NPD research.

- Assumes the role of mentor for less experienced NPD personnel.

References

ANA/NNSDO. (2010). *Nursing Professional Development Scope and Standards of Practice.* Silver Spring, MD: Authors.

Avillion, A. E. (2011). *Professional Growth in Staff Development: Strategies for New and Experienced Educators.* Danvers, MA: HCPro, Inc.

41 Competency-Based Orientation

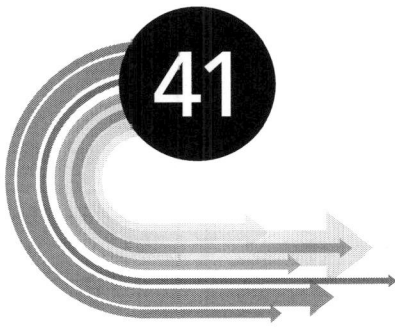

Author's note: The levels of expertise are more fully described in Chapter 38, Identifying Levels of Expertise of NPD Specialists.

Although nursing professional development (NPD) specialists are responsible for coordinating numerous aspects of nursing orientation, we often neglect to develop an adequate, competency-based orientation for newly hired NPD specialists. Just as it does with our clinical colleagues, inadequate orientation contributes to job dissatisfaction and turnover in NPD. Here are some suggestions for designing a competency-based NPD orientation based on levels of expertise (Avillion, 2011).

Preparation

Preparation for orientation is critical. The following are some tips to help with planning:

- Identify a preceptor for the new member of the NPD department. Everyone needs a preceptor, regardless of experience or role.

- Determine appropriate competencies based on level of expertise.

- Identify actions for achieving each competency.

- Identify appropriate resources to facilitate achievement of each competency.

- Identify potential political pitfalls and incorporate them into orientation. It is imperative that new employees be helped to navigate around political land mines.

- Identify people who have significant impact on the new employee's role and incorporate introductions into orientation.

- Provide information about obtaining a mentor for the new employee. Identify resources both within and outside the organization.

Sample Orientation Competency Statements

(Note that because novices are not members of the NPD department and generally function as staff nurses, NPD orientation is not addressed for the novice.)

Not every competency can be addressed within the limits of this chapter. The following competencies and actions are offered to help you design your own NPD orientation program. Competencies and action plans should be outlined before the new employee arrives and finalized in conjunction with him or her.

Advanced Beginner

Competency: Plan and implement in-service education for designated unit(s) incorporating the principles of adult learning.

Action Plan: Review principles of adult learning and how they are used in inservice design. Read Chapter 6: Principles of Adult Learning in *A Practical Guide to Staff Development* (2nd ed.) (Avillion, 2008). Work with preceptor to plan and implement an in-service education program.

Competency: Work with nursing preceptors of designated unit(s) to enhance preceptor effectiveness.

Action Plan: Under the guidance of the NPD preceptor, attend nursing preceptor training course, attend unit-specific nursing orientation, review evaluations of nursing preceptors written by orientees, review evaluations of preceptor training written by preceptors, and assist NPD specialist to analyze evaluation data.

The preceding action plan, in an actual orientation setting, would require dates for completion. Additional readings and activities would also be added. The purpose of the action plan example is to understand the need to develop and document a competency based orientation for members of the NPD department. The following are some ideas for the remaining levels of NPD expertise.

Competents

Competency: In collaboration with staff development colleagues, design needs assessment and collect needs assessment data.

Action Plan: Work with preceptor and staff development colleagues to design needs assessments. Work with preceptor to collect needs assessment data from a variety of sources. Read Chapter 10: Learning Needs Assessment in *Core Curriculum for Staff Development* (Girgenti, 2009).

Competency: Involve learners in needs assessment and identification of learning objectives.

Action Plan: Work with preceptor to meet and interact with learners and gather data pertaining to education needs. Read Chapter 14: Compiling Needs Assessment Data in *A Practical Guide to Staff Development* (2nd ed.) (Avillion, 2008).

Note that various literature resources are listed in the action plan. It is generally helpful to supply these kinds of resources for orientees.

Proficient

Competency: Gather and analyze evidence pertaining to reaction, learning, behavior, impact, and return on investment levels of evaluation.

Action Plan: Work with preceptor to gather and analyze evidence that applies to all levels of evaluation. Read *Evicence-Based Staff Development* (Avillion, 2007).

Competency: Serve as a member of designated nursing and organization committees.

Action Plan: With the assistance of preceptor, assimilate into designated committees. Attend meetings and help to identify committee data relevant to the education process.

Expert

Competency: Analyze data from committees and applies them to evidence-based practice in NPD.

Action Plan: Work with preceptor to gather and analyze relevant data. Use findings to measure the impact of education on job performance and patient outcomes. Relay findings to NPD department and others as appropriate.

Competency: Budget for NPD activities.

Action Plan: Confer with immediate supervisor on budget process and organizational priorities that influence NPD budget. Collaborate with members of the NPD department to begin to formulate budget.

Note that the expert has more sophisticated levels of competency compared to the Proficient. For example, the proficient is attending committee meetings and helping to identify relevant data as part of orientation. It is expected that an expert already has achieved this competency and is able to analyze such data independently and communicate it appropriately during orientation. Make the competencies fit the levels of expertise.

Reference

Avillion, A. E. (2011). *Professional Growth in Staff Development: Strategies for New and Experienced Educators.* Danvers, MA: HCPro, Inc.

42 Differentiating Between an Education Need and a Systems Problem

Sometimes, education can't solve a problem. This happens when lack of education isn't the issue. But how can you determine that the problem wasn't poor education or learning? Consider the following example:

Analysis of the quarterly risk management data indicates a trend in the number of patient falls occurring throughout the organization. The number has increased each month throughout the quarter and is significantly higher than last year at this time. Administration is alarmed and tells the director of nursing professional development (NPD) that he or she must implement a mandatory in-service for all direct patient care providers on fall prevention. But the first question that comes to the director's mind is, "Is the increase in falls indicative of a lack of knowledge (requiring education), or is it a systems problem?"

This type of dilemma can be particularly frustrating for NPD specialists. The reaction to bad news from risk management often provokes a knee-jerk response from leadership that involves asking for an educational endeavor that takes a great deal of time and effort on the part of educators and learners. This is worthwhile only if a true knowledge deficit exists. Otherwise, we may be overlooking the true nature of the problem. But how do we convince administration and management that more analysis is necessary before we pull every direct patient care provider away from their duties to participate in education that for most of them is redundant?

Before succumbing to a panicked request for education, propose a more thorough analysis of the problem. For example, you already know that the number of falls has increased throughout the quarter and compared to last year, the number is significantly larger. Let's analyze the problem. These questions could be applied to almost any trend in adverse occurrences, so let's use generic terminology:

- Do the adverse occurrences occur throughout the organization or are they focused on a particular unit or department?

- At what time of day or night do the events occur? Can you identify a time frame that clusters of events occur?

- What is happening when the events occur? For example, is there a pattern of occurrences during meal times, change of shifts, etc.?

- Are particular disciplines involved in the adverse events? For example, if you are analyzing medication errors, are errors traceable to nursing, pharmacy, or others?

- Have there been any changes in policies or procedures that influence the occurrence of adverse events?

- What were the consequences of the adverse events? What was the impact on patient outcomes, employee health, and organizational effectiveness?

- What, if any, were the legal ramifications of the adverse events?

- What education and/or training had been provided on topics relating to these adverse events in the past? Is there a trend between those involved in the adverse events and a lack of education and training?

- Who is involved in the analysis of the adverse occurrences? Ideally, an interdisciplinary effort is most effective. Members of the risk management committee, for instance, are logical people to participate in data analysis. The point is to focus on process not on individuals. This isn't a blame game.

> **PROFESSIONAL DEVELOPMENT ALERT**
>
> It is imperative that NPD specialists are members of organizational committees such as infection control, risk management, leadership, etc. Membership ensures access to data that may trigger education needs. The education council is also a committee that must be developed to facilitate the identification of knowledge deficits versus systems problems.

After data analysis is complete, evidence should be clarified that support (or negate) the need for education. Such evidence is also the basis of recommendations for process or systems changes. You need to be able to approach administration and management with objective findings; otherwise, it may be perceived that you are trying to escape the burden of providing education.

Ideally, the evidence you compile will help you to either trigger a much-needed change in an organizational system or processes, or identify a knowledge deficit that truly does require education.

However, there are times that, even if we show an objective need for systems change, administration and management still mandate training and education. They may be willing to investigate a change in the system, but are still convinced that education must be provided. If so, don't waste time and energy fighting a decision that is irrevocable. Instead, prepare in advance for those times when remediation education (e.g., the eight "rights" of medication administration, fall prevention, etc.) is inevitable. The following are some ideas for advance preparation:

- Identify the most common or frequent requests for remediation. Once you have accomplished this, you can prepare specific, short, concise remediation programs. You can use case studies to illustrate adherence to the eight rights of medication administration, e-mail or text blasts pertaining to infection control, etc. The idea is to plan education on topics that remain fairly consistent in content.

- Prepare a template for remediation. Such a template should include topic, learning objectives, a means for evaluating knowledge acquisition, and a means for documenting achievement of objectives. Once you have a template, create a template for each commonly identified requests for remediation. For example, for medication remediation you can include the eight rights, a brief review of the steps of proper medication administration, and data pertaining to the most common reasons for medication errors. To help the learner, include a listing of easily accessible resources to quickly identify drugs, doses, actions, and side effects.

- Work with nurse managers to develop these templates as well as a mechanism for tracking the circumstances surrounding errors and/or lack of knowledge. By tracking such circumstances, you might be able to help identify the process or systems problems that contribute to adverse events.

- Work with quality improvement and risk management committees to keep abreast of problems and how education can help alleviate such problems.

- Work with shared governance committees to identify process and systems issues and decide how to correct them.

Finally, take the initiative to objectively evaluate whether an issue is related to a knowledge deficit or a systems problem. By doing so, you can provide data to help improve organizational effectiveness and patient outcomes. If you face an irrevocable mandate to provide education, you can save yourself time and frustration by preparing in advance with the development of templates and identification of the most common requests for remediation education.

43

Business Plan and Budget Considerations

Most nursing professional development (NPD) specialists are so busy that we sometimes focus on the day-to-day budgetary processes of salaries, programming costs, and the purchase of major pieces of equipment; however, we need to remember that the budget is only one component of dealing with the business aspects of running a department. You need a comprehensive departmental business plan written from the business perspective. Such a plan helps you to gather the objective evidence you need to justify current and proposed expenses. When you meet with management and financial officers to present your budget, you need to approach it from an overall perspective of a sound business plan.

Here is an overview of the basic components of a business plan for NPD to help you not only with budget, but overall business concerns (Avillion, 2011).

Components of an NPD Business Plan

The NPD business plan has multiple components, including:

Mission Statement: This statement must clearly communicate the purpose and direction of NPD activities to people within and outside the department. It should acknowledge that departmental services are designed to improve patient/family outcomes and job performance. Figure 43.1 (available at *www.hcpro.com/downloads/10170*) offers a sample mission statement.

Vision Statement: A vision is an image that reflects your department's future and must coincide with its mission and values. A vision must be both inspiring and realistic. For example, a major medical center's NPD department may have as its vision to "be a regional leader in the provision of trauma nursing continuing education." This would not be a realistic vision for a small community hospital in a rural area.

Values Statement: A values statement is really the departmental philosophy. It describes beliefs and principles that guide departmental activities. A sample values statement is available in Figure 43.2 (available at *www.hcpro.com/downloads/10170*).

Departmental Structure and Description

You need to provide a concise description of departmental structure. A departmental organizational chart should be included as well as a brief description of departmental positions. Do not include names; include only position description, such as "five unit-based educators," "10 NPD specialists," etc.

Description is a one- or two-sentence overview of the purpose of the department, such as, "The NPD department is responsible for the orientation, in-service, and continuing education of all members of the department of nursing. NPD products and services are designed to have a positive impact on job performance and patient outcomes."

Products and Services

Provide a concise listing of the products and services you provide. This list should show that the products and services you provide are instrumental to organizational success. It doesn't have to include every program you provide, but enough to show departmental value. For example:

- Orientation for the department of nursing

- Development and evaluation of nursing preceptor program

- Evaluation, in conjunction with nursing leadership and human resources, of retention and turnover data

- Mandatory training for the organization

- Coordination of student affiliation experiences

- Semiannual regional trauma nursing educational seminars

Marketing

This section identifies how you promote your products and services. Include brief notations about internal and external advertising sources such as:

- Online in-house education calendar

- E-mail

- Smart phone "blasts"

The Path to Stress-Free Nursing Professional Development

* Direct mail for conferences

* In-house bulletin boards

Action Plan

The action plan states objectives with documentation of what actions will be taken to achieve those objectives, target dates for completion, and who has responsibility for achieving identified objectives. Figure 43.3 (available at *www.hcpro.com/downloads/10170*) is an example of a business-related action plan.

Budget

All organizations have a budget template. Your job is to complete that template using evidence from your evaluation of departmental activities. Be sure to pay attention to the following issues:

* Incorporate into salaries not only merit increases but increases that may be related to certification, obtaining graduate degrees, or other accomplishments that are linked to monetary rewards.

* When requesting funding for major equipment purchases, justify such purchases with objective data. For example, if you are requesting the purchase of simulation equipment be sure to have data available from the literature or your own simulation activities that shows how simulation improved behavior, results, etc.

* Never incorporate any budgetary item unless it is backed up by objective evidence. For instance, if you are budgeting for tuition reimbursement for an academic degree, include not only justification from hospital policy but evidence that academic preparation is associated with enhanced job performance and patient outcomes.

Executive Summary

The executive summary is written last, but is actually located as the first component of a business plan. Some administrators will read only the executive summary, which is a one- or two-page overview of your business plan. Take the first paragraph or two of each section of your plan and compile them as the executive summary. This means it is especially important to write attention-grabbing initial paragraphs of each component of your plan. Use the best, most informative pieces of information from each component to develop your executive summary.

Reference

Avillion, A. E. (2011). *The Survival of Staff Development: Measure Outcomes and Demonstrate Value to Establish an Indispensable Department.* Danvers, MA: HCPro, Inc.

44

Shared Governance

Shared governance is an organizational management model that is based on shared decision-making or shared leadership. Reported outcomes of shared governance include increased retention, decreased turnover, increased job satisfaction, decreased length of patient stay, and improved patient outcomes (Swihart, 2011). The American Nurses Credentialing Center Magnet Recognition Program® (MRP)reflects the values and process of shared governance. It is no wonder that organizations striving to attain or maintain MRP status have embraced shared governance.

All shared governance models support the principle that the nursing staff are responsible and accountable for, and have authority over, all decisions related to professional nursing practice (Swihart, 2011).

It is not possible to describe the shared governance implementation process in a short chapter. What is presented is a description of essential councils and their importance, according to Swihart (2011), which is also an excellent, detailed resource for planning and implementing your own shared governance model.

Overview of Councils

Much of the work of shared governance is accomplished by councils. The first step in council formulation is to identify desired outcomes. Once the outcomes are known, councils can be initiated. Different councils have different purposes:

- **Leadership council (also called management or coordinating council):** Its purpose is to provide guidance and linkage to the governing councils and act as a resource for the nurse executive, nurse leaders, and nurse managers to become involved in activities related to the provision of nursing care at point of service.

- **Unit-level councils:** Unit-level councils are the core structure for implementation of shared governance. It is at this level that direct patient care providers have an opportunity to share in the decision-making process and determine outcomes specific to the needs of each particular unit.

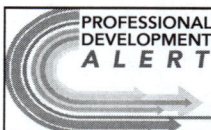

PROFESSIONAL DEVELOPMENT ALERT

With shared decision-making comes change, responsibility, and accountability. Nurses need support as they assume responsibility for decisions and activities that once may have been purely managerial responsibilities.

- **Practice council:** This council sets the criteria for evidence-based practice (EBP) that is consistent with professional standards of practice. This council selects a theoretical base for practice, sets practice and performance standards, and defines career advancement.

- **Quality council:** This council monitors and evaluates performance and outcome measurements based on EBP, research findings, and the best practice evidence available. It provides a mechanism for interdisciplinary collaboration to improve patient outcomes.

- **Nursing professional development council (sometimes called an education council):** This council provides and oversees orientation, assesses ongoing learning and competency needs, and ensures professional competency and professional growth and development via in-service, continuing education, and other education-related activities.

Council Membership

It's important to understand what it means to be a council member and what the role and responsibilities of a council member are. The following should be included in the description and explanation of a council member:

- Council members speak on behalf of the groups they represent. Some organizations ask persons to apply for council membership. Others actually elect representatives.

- Council members will be assigned to various tasks and responsibilities. They need to be allotted time to work on these assignments as time would be allotted for any other work responsibility.

- It is recommended that 70% to 90% of council members be direct patient care providers.

- It is generally recommended that councils be composed of between seven to 15 members at a time.

- Two year terms of service are recommended.

- The council meeting times depends on the needs of the members and the work to be accomplished. Some organizations prefer that councils meet for eight hours once per month. Members may attend meetings via phone or web. By having an entire work day devoted to the meeting, plans can be made in advance for patient coverage.

Shared governance fosters empowerment and commitment from an organization's employees. It helps to identify best practices and promote desired patient outcomes and job satisfaction.

Reference

Swihart, D. (2011). *Shared Governance: A Practical Approach to Transform Professional Nursing Practice* (2nd ed.). Danvers, MA: HCPro., Inc.

45

Copyright Concerns

Kate is the nursing professional development (NPD) specialist for pediatrics in a large community hospital. As part of a regional conference on the psychosocial impact of chronic diseases/disorders in children, she is addressing the problems, both physical and psychosocial, of stuttering. Kate decides to show several short clips from the movie *The King's Speech*, which deals with the late King George VI of England's efforts to conquer his own stuttering as an adult. The movie clips are brief, and in total take up no more than 10 minutes of presentation time. However, the day after the conference, Kate is summoned to the vice president of nursing's office. The vice president has heard about Kate's use of the movie clips and is quite concerned that Kate has violated copyright laws and may have made the hospital vulnerable to a fine for copyright infringement.

Introduction

Copyright is the "author's or owner's right to have control over copying an original work, including the right to copy, distribute, and adapt the work" (Puetz, 2010). Violation or infringement of copyright laws is a matter of some concern to all NPD specialists. Unfortunately, there are no absolutes when it comes to the legalities of copyright. The information in this section is not intended as legal advice. For specific, reliable answers to copyright concerns, consult with your organization's legal counsel and utilize the U.S. Copyright Office's website for detailed information (*www.copyright.gov*). Still, there are some guidelines we can use to avoid or at least reduce the risk of copyright violation.

First, you need to know that your work (or someone else's work) is protected under copyright the minute it is created and put in a tangible form that can be seen or accessed with the aid of a machine or device (Puetz, 2010). This means that the work cannot be copied in part or in entirety without permission. Copyright lasts for a specific period of time, after which (unless the work is copyrighted again) the work becomes part of the public domain and can be copied without permission.

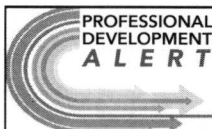

> **PROFESSIONAL DEVELOPMENT ALERT**
>
> Different kinds of work are copyrighted for different lengths of time. To find out what the time frames are for different kinds of work, visit *www.copyright.gov/help/faq*.

Types of Works Protected by Copyright

Works protected by copyright include (U.S. Copyright Office, 2006):

- Literary works

- Musical works including words that may accompany the music

- Pictorial, graphic, and sculptural works

- Dramatic works including any music that accompanies the work

- Sound recordings

- Motion pictures, videos, DVDs, photographs, cartoons, and other audiovisual works

- Architectural works

- Pantomimes and choreographic works

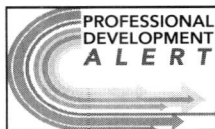

> **PROFESSIONAL DEVELOPMENT ALERT** — Remember that work published on the Internet is also protected by copyright laws.

What Cannot Be Copyrighted

The following cannot be copyrighted (Puetz, 2010; U.S. Copyright Office, 2006):

- Work that is not in a tangible format such as a verbal lecture that is not recorded, written down, or saved electronically.

- Facts, ideas, titles, and names. (e.g., "George Washington was the first President of the United States").

- Works that are entirely made up of information that is common knowledge and have no original authorship (e.g., "The Twin Towers of the World Trade Center collapsed on September 11, 2001").

- Blank forms such as a blank template.

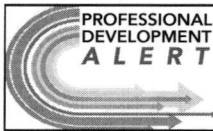

> **PROFESSIONAL DEVELOPMENT ALERT**
>
> Although the preceding items cannot be copyrighted they may be protected by patents and trademarks. A patent protects inventions and discoveries, and a trademark protects words, symbols, or designs that identify a person or group (Puetz, 2010).

Fair Use

Fair use is "the allowable use of limited amounts of a copyrighted work for the purpose of criticism, news, teaching, scholarship, or research without getting permission from the copyright holder" (Puetz, 2010). Some NPD specialists believe that if they are copying and distributing an article for use in an education program there is no danger of copyright violation. This is seldom true. It is always better to apply for permission to reprint an article than take the chance of copyright infringement. It is better to pay for the cost of reprinting an article, for example, than pay for copyright infringement. Up to $150,000 can be charged for each work if the copyright owner can prove willful infringement. Additional costs may be for statutory damages and attorney's fees (Puetz, 2010).

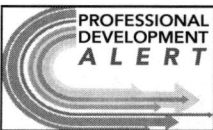

> **PROFESSIONAL DEVELOPMENT ALERT**
>
> Remember to reference any scholarly work meticulously. Many NPD specialists publish in journals and books. Be sure to cite your references carefully.

Copyright Checklist

To help you determine what questions to ask when including copyrighted material in your own work, Figure 45.1 (available at *www.hcpro.com/downloads/10170*) is a checklist developed by Puetz (2010).

References

Puetz, L. R. (2010). Copyright and fair use. In Avillion A. E. *Innovation in Nursing Staff Development: Teaching Strategies to Enhance Learner Outcomes.* (pp. 117-132). Danvers, MA: HCPro, Inc.

U. S. Copyright Office. (2006). Copyright in general. Retrieved February 3, 2012, from *www.copyright.gov/help/faq/faq-general. html#protect*.

46   Ethical Issues

Ethics are the moral principles that guide our behaviors. Nurses function under the auspices of various codes of behavior such as Nurse Practice Acts, The Florence Nightingale Pledge, The American Nurses Association Code of Ethics, and the principles espoused by various professional associations.

Most nursing ethics codes note that:

- Nurses must treat patients with compassion and respect regardless of their social or economic status, race, culture, religion, personal characteristics, their personal decisions about their healthcare, or the nature of their health problems.

- Nurses' primary commitment is to the patient (whether an individual, family, or community).

- Nurses have a duty to maintain confidentiality of all patient information.

- Nurses collaborate with other healthcare professionals and the community to meet health needs.

- Nurses are responsible for their own individual practice.

- Nurses participate in maintaining and improving healthcare services.

- Nurses participate in the advancement of their profession.

(Bosek & Savage, 2007)

The preceding list is not all-inclusive but summarizes the highlights of our ethical responsibilities as nurses. As nursing professional development (NPD) specialists, we also have ethical responsibilities to our learners. NPD specialists:

- Must treat learners with compassion and respect regardless of social or economic status, race, culture, religion, personal characteristics.

- Are committed to the well-being of patients and the professional growth and development of learners.

- Have a duty to maintain confidentiality of learning outcomes unless those outcomes relate to patient safety.

- Collaborate with learners to design education and training that enhance job performance and organizational effectiveness.

NPD-Specific Ethical Dilemmas

The preceding statements are not all-inclusive but are critical to the ethics of our specialty. Although we often consider the ethical implications of direct patient care, we sometimes forget that NPD has its own particular set of ethical responsibilities, as well as dilemmas. The following are some examples of NPD ethical dilemmas and possible strategies to resolve them.

Example 1: Falsified qualifications

During orientation a newly hired cardiac critical care nurse is able to challenge several aspects of orientation (a cardiac pharmacology exam, arrhythmia interpretation course, and emergency simulation exercises) by successfully passing post-test written exams and psychomotor skill demonstrations. These successes mean that she does not have to take the formal orientation classes on these subjects. One of the prerequisites for challenging portions of critical care orientation is that the candidate must have at least two years of cardiac critical care. Several weeks after the new nurse begins to work on the unit with a preceptor, you discover that she has falsified her qualifications and has less than six months prior experience as a cardiac critical care nurse. Her preceptor is pleased with her progress and her coworkers speak highly of her. What should you do?

You may be tempted to do nothing. After all, she passed her exams and skill demonstration and is doing well on the unit. Ethically, however, you have an obligation to report this to her nurse manager. She did lie about qualifications, which poses the concern that she may be capable of lying about other issues. Although you have a duty to the learner, your primary obligation is to the patients on the unit. Additionally, if you allow one nurse who does not meet prerequisites to challenge portions of orientation, you must allow others to do so as well. You would also need to change the standards of certain aspects of orientation. Finally, remember that the new nurse has violated ethical standards as well by lying to you.

Example 2: Pressure to falsify documentation

The organization's written policy states that all employees, including administrative staff, must attend annual mandatory training in such topics as safety, disaster preparedness, etc. The CEO and his administrative assistant routinely avoid such training. The Joint Commission surveyors have now arrived for an unannounced survey. The CEO tells you to document that he and his assistant attended the training last month. What do you do?

You are being asked to falsify records. You can offer to review the information with both the CEO and his assistant and document today's date. What you should not do is lie and sign your name to a false document. Ask yourself if the CEO would be willing to falsify records for you! This is a very difficult ethical dilemma that is, sadly, not uncommon. If you falsify records and this falsification is discovered, your professional credibility is destroyed. You may need to try to avoid this dilemma by bringing training directly to the CEO in his or her office. You also need to enlist the support of your immediate supervisor in resolving these kinds of dilemmas.

Example 3: Exam cheating

An online course concerning pathophysiology of spinal cord injury is mandatory for all nurses working on the neurological rehabilitation unit. Your pleasure at the high post-test examination scores is ruined when you find that one of the nurses has hacked into the answer database and has posted questions and answers on her Facebook page. What do you do?

Social media helps spread information quickly to a great number of people. Unfortunately, this can make it a breeding ground for ethical dilemmas. You need to report this activity to the nurse's nurse manager. You also need to rewrite the exams and have all nurses who took the exam prior to this discovery retake the exam. This will certainly not make you popular. However, you have an ethical obligation to ensure, as far as possible, that knowledge is actually being acquired, not obtained by cheating.

Reference

Bosek, M. S. DeWolf, & Savage, T. A. (2007). *The Ethical Component of Nursing Education: Integrating Ethics into Clinical Experience.* Philadelphia: Lippincott Williams & Wilkins.

47

Legal Issues

Education designed to help the healthcare community avoid legal pitfalls is primarily directed toward those who provide direct patient care. However, those of us who work in nursing professional development (NPD) are becoming more aware of our own vulnerability when it comes to legal action. We have a legal duty to our learners and, indirectly, to the patients our learners will care for.

Nursing malpractice is a violation of professional duty manifested as a failure to meet a standard of care or a failure to use knowledge or skills that another similarly educated and trained nurse would use in similar circumstances (Doyle, 2009). In order to be liable for malpractice, four elements must be shown: duty owed to the patient, breach of duty owed to the patient, injury, and causation (Doyle, 2009).

How do these elements affect NPD specialists? Most of us do not provide direct patient care or only do so on an occasional basis. Our primary responsibilities are those of education and training. However, these responsibilities require that we fulfill our duties to learners (and indirectly to patients) in such a manner that we avoid the elements of malpractice. It is important that we help our NPD colleagues to understand that we have very particular legal obligations. Let's look at each of these elements in relation to NPD practice.

Duty to Learners

This section is called "duty to learners" not "duty to patients." Although "duty owed to patient" is the first of the four elements that make us vulnerable to malpractice, our roles as NPD specialists means we are more likely to face legal consequences if we fail to fulfill our responsibilities to our learners; however, it's important to remember that this does not negate our responsibilities as nurses to patients. Duty is established as soon as we begin assessment of learning needs. All aspects of the education process are subject to a scrutiny of how well we fulfill our duty to learners. We must be able to document that we have assessed learning needs and, after prioritizing those needs based on organizational goals and patient populations, have developed education to meet those needs.

The Path to Stress-Free Nursing Professional Development

We must show that evaluation is performed to determine not only learner satisfaction, but to measure the impact of education on job performance and organizational effectiveness. Documentation must show how we review and revise education based on evidence acquired from evaluations as well as advances and changes in the delivery of healthcare. In other words, it is our duty to provide learners with the education and training they need and to make sure that such education and training is timely, accessible, and effective.

Breach of Duty

Breach of duty, for NPD practice, means that we have failed to plan and deliver education and training that meets identified needs. This failure could involve, for example, inaccuracies in content, inadequate assessment of learner competency, or failure to provide a safe environment for learners. A breach of duty could result in a learner delivering substandard care to a patient. If this occurs, we could be held partially responsible for errors made as a result of failing to meet our duty as educators. Failure to provide a safe environment may make us liable for injury to a learner. Suppose we are teaching nurses how to safely transfer spinal cord injured patients from bed to wheelchair, but do not provide sufficient instruction or do not monitor the learner's ability to perform the transfer without injury. If the learner is injured while lifting the patient, we could be held accountable for his or her injury.

Injury

In order to be held liable for malpractice, the learner or patient must prove that injury occurred. Suppose a NPD specialist relays incorrect information about a new cardiac drug to be administered in an emergency situation. As a result of this information, a nurse administers the drug incorrectly, and the patient suffers a serious adverse reaction. The NPD specialist could also be held, in part, responsible since he or she provided learners with incorrect information.

Causation

Proving causation requires that the patient or learner prove that injury is caused by the breach of duty. This means that what the NPD specialist did or failed to do caused injury. Consider the preceding example. Incorrect information was part of an education program. A nurse, relying on the accuracy of the information received as part of continuing education efforts, administered a cardiac drug incorrectly. The patient suffered injury as a result of this error. Cause can be traced from failure to provide accurate and appropriate education to the nurse who made the medication error based on misinformation.

Tips for Meeting NPD Legal Responsibilities

NPD specialists have a legal responsibility to provide accurate and timely information and in-service, as well as to assess how well learners achieve learning objectives and intervene if they are not met. The following are some issues to address when considering these legal responsibilities:

- Document and prioritize needs assessment data in correlation with organizational goals and objectives and patient populations served.

- Make sure that learning objectives are explicit.

- Ensure that adequate evaluation takes place to measure the achievement of learning objectives.

- Make sure that education content is accurate and timely.

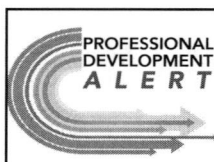

> **PROFESSIONAL DEVELOPMENT ALERT**
>
> If an error in education content is discovered make sure that it is corrected as soon as it is discovered. Make sure that all learners who received this information are notified personally (e.g., e-mail, PDA, etc.) and that corrections are posted as appropriate on the NPD section of the organization's employee website.

- Document how evaluation data are used to revise and plan education.

- Educate all members of the NPD department regarding legal implications for NPD practice.

Critical Thinking Exercises

Think about using some critical thinking exercises as part of the continuing legal education for NPD specialists. The following are some sample exercises.

Exercise 1

Martin is the NPD specialist responsible for the continuing education and in-service of the physical rehabilitation units located within a large 1,500-bed medical center. He is providing in-service and continuing education for nurses new to the stroke rehabilitation unit. Part of his teaching involves teaching these nurses to safely transfer patients from bed to wheelchair and wheelchair to toilet. One of the nurses, Kathy, fails to achieve competency on return demonstration. Martin and Kathy identify remediation tactics and he documents that Kathy is not cleared to perform transfers independently. Both he and Kathy sign the competency form that states Kathy is not to perform transfers without assistance. Kathy returns to the unit and proceeds to transfer a patient from his bed to a wheelchair without assistance. The patient falls and breaks a leg. Answer the following questions:

1. Have the four elements of malpractice been met?

2. Have these four elements been met by Martin's behavior or Kathy's behavior or both of them?

3. How could patient injury have been prevented?

The Path to Stress-Free Nursing Professional Development

Exercise 2

Maria is a critical care nurse who has worked in the emergency department for many years. She is required to achieve and maintain Advanced Cardiac Life Support (ACLS) certification. However, when she takes the written component of the exam she fails to achieve a passing score. Maria explains to Monica the NPD specialist responsible for ACLS training, that she is in the middle of a nasty divorce and is having difficulty concentrating. Hospital policy is that failure to pass any component of the ACLS training results in suspension from work until certification is achieved. Maria asks Monica to delay reporting the results until she can retake the exam. Monica agrees to do so. Later that day Maria makes a serious medication error during a code in the emergency department. Information related to the medication was included in the exam that Maria failed. The patient suffered an adverse reaction but was successfully resuscitated. However, the patient's family is taking about filing a lawsuit. Maria, when discussing the incident with her supervisor, blames Monica for the error. "She knew I failed the exam, but told me I could work anyway. It's her fault, not mine."

Address these issues.

1. Explain if the four elements of malpractice have been met.
2. Explain who is liable for the patient's injury and why.
3. Discuss what actions Maria should have taken in this situation.
4. Discuss what actions Monica should have taken in this situation.

Exercise 3

Denise is teaching a physical assessment course using equipment that simulates abnormal heart and lung sounds. One of the learners is concerned that the equipment is incorrectly plugged into electrical outlets via several extension cords. Denise has only a limited amount of time to teach the course and tells the nurse that "there is no danger." The learner suffers an electric shock and is burned when using the simulation equipment. The burn causes her to lose several days of work. The learner is talking about suing Denise.

1. Did Denise's actions meet the four elements of malpractice? Why or why not?
2. Did Denise have a duty to ensure that the simulation equipment was safe to use?
3. What actions could have been taken to avoid the adverse outcomes of this situation?

Reference

Doyle, R. (2009). *Evidence-based Nursing Guide to Legal & Professional Issues*. Philadelphia: Wolters Kluwer Health/Lippincott Williams & Wilkins.

48

Institute of Medicine Implications for Nursing Professional Development

In October 2010, the Institute of Medicine (IOM) published *The Future of Nursing: Advancing Health* (IOM, 2010). This publication is the result of two years of study and research conducted by the IOM and the Robert Wood Johnson Foundation. People who participated in the project listened to testimony about the current state of nursing practice and the nursing profession's potential impact on current efforts to enhance and improve healthcare delivery in the United States, reviewed the literature about the state of nursing practice, and visited a variety of healthcare facilities to gain insight into nurses and their practice.

At the conclusion of their efforts, participants reported four critical messages (IOM, 2010; Yoder-Wise & Esquibel, 2011):

- Nurses should practice to the "full" extent of their education and training.

- Nurses should attain higher levels of education and training.

- Nurses should be equal partners with other healthcare professionals in the redesign of the ways in which healthcare is offered in the United States.

- Nurses and other healthcare professionals must improve data collection and work to improve healthcare organizations' information infrastructure.

IOM researchers identified eight recommendations (IOM, 2010; Yoder-Wise, 2011):

- Remove barriers to the scope of nursing practice.

- Increase opportunities for nurses to lead and implement collaborative improvement activities.

- Implement nurse residency programs.

- Increase the number of nurses who have baccalaureate degrees to 80% by 2020.

- Double the nurses who possess doctorates by 2020.

- Make certain that nurses engage in lifelong learning.

- Educate and enable nurses to lead change initiatives to advance health.

- Establish an infrastructure that encourages and enables the collection and analysis of interprofessional healthcare workforce data.

These messages and recommendations have significant implications for the practice of NPD. Many of these ideas (such as nurse residency programs and lifelong learning) have long been espoused by NPD specialists. It is now critical that we take the information from this report and use it to justify a number of initiatives including:

- Collaborate with nursing leadership to design and implement nurse residency programs.

- Collaborate with nursing leadership, interdisciplinary leadership, and administration to facilitate career advancement programs for nurses so that they may practice to the full extent of their education and training.

- Review and revise preceptor programs with an emphasis on increasing retention and decreasing turnover.

- Advocate for tuition reimbursement for the pursuit of baccalaureate and graduate degrees.

- Increase opportunities for staff nurses to become members of both nursing and housewide committees and task forces so that they become equal partners in the redesign of healthcare delivery.

- Offer opportunities for nurses pursuing baccalaureate and graduate degrees to work with NPD specialists as they work on clinical and research projects related to their academic pursuits.

- Develop and implement leadership education to prepare nurses to assume leadership roles in healthcare organization.

- Offer continuing education pertaining to healthcare reform.

- Facilitate data collection as it pertains to research, healthcare delivery, and evidence-based practice.

- Support legislation that enables RNs to practice to the full extent of their education and training.

- Offer education and training and in the form of technology "blasts" (e.g., texts, e-mails, etc.) that help nurses comprehend healthcare reform and legislation that affects healthcare in general and nursing practice in particular.

References

Institute of Medicine (IOM). (2010). *The Future of Nursing: Leading Change/Advancing Health*. Washington, DC: Author.

Yoder-Wise, P. I., & Esquibel, K. A. (2011). The future of nursing and continuing education. *The Journal of Continuing Education in Nursing*, 42(3), 99-100.

49 Institute of Safe Medication Practices Implications for Nursing Professional Development

Nursing professional development (NPD) specialists are involved in assessing and helping to improve safe medication practices on an almost daily basis. We are (or should be) constantly on the lookout for resources to help us with this responsibility. One invaluable resource is the Institute of Safe Medication Practices (ISMP).

ISMP is a nonprofit organization designed to educate the healthcare community as well as consumers about safe medication practices. Its website is a treasure-trove of information *(www.ismp.org)*. Here are some ideas for making the most of the ISMP as a professional development resource:

- Just as with The Joint Commission, someone from the NPD department should assume the responsibility for perusing the ISMP website for the latest information about its research findings, tools, education resources, and newsletters. The information should be synthesized for use in NPD activities.

- Participate, as appropriate, in ISMP online surveys. These surveys are a good way of gathering data from national sources.

- Use the ISMP's list of high-alert medications, error-prone abbreviation list, "do not crush" list, and other tools as part of your education efforts pertaining to safe medication practices.

- Review the continuing education programs offered by the ISMP. Consider budgeting attendance to at least one program into your NPD budget.

- Participate in the ISMP self-assessment opportunities (click on the link under Education & Awareness on the website's home page).

- Review the listing of consumer resources. These are helpful not only for patient education but as a mechanism for professional development activities as well.

- Review the descriptions of the ISMP newsletters. Some are available without a charge, such as the newsletter for consumers.

The ISMP is an excellent resource for healthcare professionals. It can provide NPD specialists with significant resources for education and training.

50

Keeping Up With
The Joint Commission

Joint Commission preparedness is an ongoing concern. Although there are no easy ways to keep up with the multitude of Joint Commission data that are generated almost daily, there are ways to simplify the process. The following are some suggestions for streamlining Joint Commission readiness from a professional development perspective:

- Ensure that a member of the nursing professional development (NPD) department is a member of the Joint Commission preparedness committee or task force. Most organizations have such a committee and it is imperative that NPD is represented. This way you will be able to identify education needs and work with interdisciplinary colleagues to ensure that they are met.

- Assign one NPD specialist to be the point person for Joint Commission assessment. This is the person who reviews the Joint Commission resources for education resources, changes to standards, etc. Thanks to the Joint Commission website, this type of information is easily accessed.

- Subscribe to The Joint Commission online. This is a free service and you can sign up at the Joint Commission's website (*www.jointcommission.org*). This is a weekly e-newsletter. You'll receive an e-mail alert advising you that the latest edition is ready for viewing. It covers everything from regulation updates to new education resources to patient education information. It is an invaluable resource.

- Access the Joint Commission's Targeted Solutions Tool™ (TST). This is a unique online application tool designed to help accredited facilities resolve some of the most common quality and safety issues. The TST helps users to assess their actual performance and identify barriers to achieving excellence. The tool then offers solutions that are customized to help them deal with their particular problems. The TST initially provided information on hand hygiene compliance, but is being expanded to include a variety of other Center projects, including enhancing the accuracy of hand-off communications, reducing wrong-site surgery risk, and dealing with the challenge of surgical site infections. Further information is available on the Joint Commission website. Type Targeted Solution Tool into the search box on the website's home page or contact John Cullinan at *jcullinan@jointcommission.org*.

- Avoid bombarding staff with too many Joint Commission updates. Weekly e-blasts may cause staff members to "tune out" this type of excessive communications. Sharing via e-blasts is okay, but limit it to critical information. Don't just repeat information published by The Joint Commission. Make changes or new endeavors applicable by inventing a hypothetical clinical scenario and show how the new information affects patient care. For example, introduce a new patient education tool by developing a clinical scenario and showing how the tool will help both patients and caregivers.

- Continue or initiate mock surveys on all shifts and include weekends. Involve members of the management and administrative team in role playing various scenarios. They could portray surveyors, patients, visitors, etc.

- Use all types media to share Joint Commission information. Don't limit yourself to technology "blasts" such as e-mail and the organization's employee section of its website. Use bulletin boards and mandatory training. Incorporate examples of Joint Commission standards in all type of education. For instance, a class on demonstrating physical assessment could also include charting standards, confidentiality issues, etc.

- Finally, do take advantage of the variety of free resources that can be downloaded on the Joint Commission's website. Encourage the NPD point person to pay special attention to these resources and share them with colleagues during NPD staff meetings and committee meetings as appropriate.

Facilitating Joint Commission accreditation is an important aspect of NPD practice. Remain constantly alert to any changes in education requirements and ensure Joint Commission preparedness discussions are a regular part of NPD staff meetings.

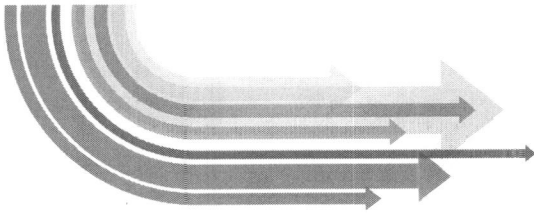

Nursing Education Instructional Guide

Target Audience

Staff development specialists

Unit educators

Nurse managers and leaders

Chief nursing officers/chief nursing executives

Directors of nursing

Vice presidents of nursing

Clinical nurse leaders

Advanced practice nurses

Charge nurses

Retention coordinators

Staff nurses

Statement of Need

This book provides strategies on providing efficient and effective nursing professional development.

Faculty

Adrianne E. Avillion, DEd, RN, is the owner of Avillion's Curriculum Design in York, PA, and specializes in designing continuing education programs for healthcare professionals and freelance medical writing. She is the editor of the e-newsletter *Staff Development Weekly* and is a frequent presenter at various conferences and conventions devoted to continuing education and professional development. She is the author of *Evidence-Based Staff Development: Strategies to Create, Measure, and Refine Your Program; A Practical Guide to Staff Development: Evidence-Based Tools and Techniques for Effective Education*, Second Edition; and *The Survival of Staff Development: Measure Outcomes and Demonstrate Value to Establish an Indispensable Department*.

Contributing author **Barbara A. Brunt, MA, MN, RN-BC, NE-BC,** is director of nursing education and staff development for Summa Health System in Akron, OH. Brunt is currently serving a two-year term as president of NNSDO. She has held a variety of staff development positions, including education coordinator and director, for the past 30 years. Brunt has presented on a variety of topics both locally and nationally and has published numerous articles, chapters, and books. She is a noted author, including *Competencies for Staff Educators: Tools to Evaluate and Enhance Nursing Professional Development*, published by HCPro.

Continuing Education

Nursing Contact Hours:

HCPro, Inc., is accredited as a provider of continuing nursing education by the American Nurses Credentialing Center's Commission on Accreditation.

This educational activity for three nursing contact hours is provided by HCPro, Inc.

Faculty Disclosure Statement

HCPro, Inc., has confirmed that none of the faculty, contributors, or planners have any relevant financial relationships to disclose related to the content of this educational activity.

Disclosure of Unlabeled Use

This educational activity may contain discussion of published and/or investigational uses of agents that are not indicated by the U.S. Food and Drug Administration. HCPro, Inc., does not recommend the use of any agent outside of the labeled indications. The opinions expressed in the educational activity are those of the faculty and do not necessarily represent the views of HCPro, Inc. Please refer to the official prescribing information for each product for discussion of approved indications, contraindications, and warnings.

Non-Endorsement of Products

Accreditation of this educational program does not imply endorsement by the American Nurses Credentialing Center or HCPro, Inc., of any products displayed in conjunction with this activity.

Instructions

In order to be eligible to receive your nursing contact hours or physician continuing education credits for this activity, you are required to do the following:

1. Read the book, *The Path to Stress-Free Nursing Professional Development: 50 No-Nonsense Solutions to Everyday Challenges*

2. Go online to: *www.hcpro.com/stressfreenursing/e1*

3. Complete the exam and receive a passing score of 80% or higher

4. Complete the evaluation

5. Provide your contact information on the exam and evaluation

A certificate will be e-mailed to you immediately following your successful completion of the quiz.

NOTE:

This book and associated exam are intended for individual use only. If you would like to provide this continuing education exam to other members of your nursing or physician staff, please contact our customer service department at 877-727-1728 to place your order. The exam fee schedule is as follows:

Exam Quantity	Fee
1	$0
2 – 25	$15 per person
26 – 50	$12 per person
51 – 100	$8 per person
101+	$5 per person